# MODERN PSYCHEDELICS

**ALSO BY JOE DOLCE**

*Brave New Weed: Adventures into the Uncharted World of Cannabis*

# MODERN PSYCHEDELICS

## THE HANDBOOK FOR MINDFUL EXPLORATION

## JOE DOLCE

### FOREWORD BY JULIE HOLLAND, MD

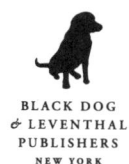

BLACK DOG
& LEVENTHAL
PUBLISHERS
NEW YORK

Black Dog & Leventhal Publishers
Hachette Book Group
1290 Avenue of the Americas, New York, NY 10104
www.blackdogandleventhal.com

 BlackDogandLeventhal  @BDLev

First Edition: August 2025

Published by Black Dog & Leventhal Publishers, an imprint of Hachette Book Group, Inc.
The Black Dog & Leventhal Publishers name and logo are trademarks of Hachette Book Group, Inc.

Black Dog & Leventhal books may be purchased in bulk for business, educational, or promotional use. For more information, please contact your local bookseller or the Hachette Book Group Special Markets Department at Special.Markets@hbgusa.com.

The publisher is not responsible for websites (or their content) that are not owned by the publisher.

Print book cover design by Aaron Lowell Denton
Print book interior design by Sheryl Kober

Library of Congress Cataloging-in-Publication Data
Names: Dolce, Joe (periodical editor), author.
Title: Modern psychedelics: a handbook for skillful use / Joe Dolce ;
  foreword by Julie Holland.
Description: First edition. | New York, NY: Black Dog & Leventhal
  Publishers, [2025] | Includes bibliographical references and index. |
  Summary: "A complete, user-friendly, evidence-based, up-to-the-minute handbook for adults who are interested in microdosing and the skillful use of psychedelics, including LSD, magic mushrooms/psilocybin, ketamine, DMT, ayahuasca, MDMA, and mescaline/peyote"—Provided by publisher.
Identifiers: LCCN 2024029860 (print) | LCCN 2024029861 (ebook) |
  ISBN 9780762488537 (paperback) | ISBN 9780762488544 (ebook)
Subjects: LCSH: Hallucinogenic drugs. | Hallucinogenic drugs—Therapeutic
  use.
Classification: LCC RM324.8 .D65 2025 (print) | LCC RM324.8 (ebook) | DDC
  615.7/883—dc23/eng/20241120
LC record available at https://lccn.loc.gov/2024029860
LC ebook record available at https://lccn.loc.gov/2024029861

ISBNs: 978-0-7624-8853-7 (trade paperback); 978-0-7624-8854-4 (ebook)

Printed in the United States of America

LSC-C

Printing 1, 2025

# Contents

--------------------------------

No—no words—no words to describe it. Poetry!
They should have sent a poet. So beautiful.
So beautiful. I had no idea.

CARL SAGAN, *Contact*

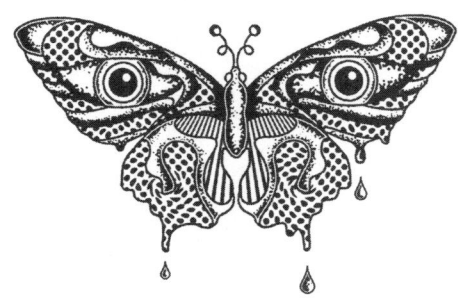

# Foreword

Cliché as it may seem, one of my earliest LSD experiences was during my first year of college. The Grateful Dead were in town, playing at a stadium in Philadelphia within walking distance of campus, and there was plenty of low-priced quality blotter available in the parking lot for whoever would like. (This is how things were in the 1980s, friends. Acid aplenty.)

Forty years later, the memories of the show are patchy, but I know the night felt like it would go on forever. My freshman roommates and I walked home on what seemed like a giant treadmill. Once back at our dorm, the decision of what to do next felt overwhelming.

My friend began insisting that she was not capable of any cognitive processing, pleading with us to understand this basic fact about her experience: "I don't know anything! I never knew anything!" (Needless to say, this quote stayed in our friend-group lexicon for years.)

The Don't-Know Mind she had discovered on LSD is an ideal state of existence in Buddhist philosophy, allowing presence and openness. Part of the drag of being an adult is that our waking consciousness becomes one of "been there, done that." On a neurological level, that's known as relying on our priors. Obliterating our previous assumptions allows us to see life with fresh eyes and fresh minds. Many of us are rediscovering, as adults, what we first saw as children, with the help of psychedelics.

This ability to view anything from a different perspective—getting *un*used to something you're used to—creates entrancing novelty. Variety may be the spice of life, but for some of us, it is more of a staple. We are the few, the proud, the psychonauts. If you're not one of us, this book will help you catch up quickly, to learn some of what we've figured out so far.

Are we willing to boldly go where we've not gone before, to examine not only the intricacies of a flower but also our own inner worlds and galaxies? Are these formative experiences of our adolescence actually the "childish things" that we are meant to put aside as adults? Or can we integrate the visions and wisdom of youth into adult life?

Working, relaxing, talking to your lover . . . there's a psychedelic for that. (And even though Joe doesn't include the most common, desacralized, and disrespected psychedelic, cannabis, in this book, let us not forget its enormous value. You can learn more about that in his previous book, *Brave New Weed*.)

With so many new drugs, new drug policies, and the handy guidebook you're holding, we are lucky to be living with such abundance. Likewise, this is an amazing time to be a psychiatrist. We've never had so many new medications to explore. The field of psychopharmacology had been stagnant for decades—the daily-dose approach to correct a "chemical imbalance" barely beats a placebo or a walk in the woods. With ketamine-assisted therapy available nationwide, people are getting used to the idea that a medicine can be helpful even though it's not administered every day, and that we can participate in the work ourselves, inside.

Psychedelic medicines are powerful. They can remodel a person's perspective and behavior. In a perfect world, they will not only help to change us as individuals, but they may also change how medicine is delivered; they will eventually transform psychiatry, neurology, rehabilitative medicine, and end-of-life care.

As I write this, there are wars, famine, fires, floods, and the very real threat of authoritarianism. We are watching our civil rights eroding in real time. Amid a background of political uncertainty and polarization, socioeconomic inequity and injustice, we are increasingly feeling fear and powerlessness. Our electronically connected lives allow us to experience terror and trauma far from our homes, while we are physically disconnected from ourselves, our communities, and the natural world that surrounds us.

These constant onslaughts are a lot to carry, and it's no wonder so many of us opt to lay our burdens down and disappear into a dissociative concoction of deeper electronic distraction and other "drugs of abuse." It's also no wonder that rates of depression, anxiety, addiction, and particularly suicide are climbing. As access to traditional medical care is getting increasingly challenging, more people are experimenting with an alternative approach to treating their own fear, anxiety, and PTSD.

This approach is being bolstered by the research. Psilocybin reliably induces a mystical state, which correlates with the efficacy of the experience. MDMA can work for some veterans with PTSD. Ibogaine research and treatments, particularly with added magnesium, are being conducted to treat opioid addiction. And microdosing LSD shows promise for everyone from tech bros to your grandmother.

Two psychedelic conferences (the Multidisciplinary Association for Psychedelic Studies [MAPS] meeting in Denver in June 2023, and Horizons in New York City in May 2024) felt like the high-water marks of hype and optimism. Unfortunately, in the summer of 2024, the FDA declined to approve MDMA with psychotherapy as a treatment for PTSD. That was a gut punch for many of us that we're still processing. More recently, the timetable for FDA approval of psilocybin with supportive therapy has been pushed back by a year or more.

We've come far, and the research is convincing, but it's not simple, and we'll clearly have to wait longer than we originally thought. It's like the psychedelic community is now arriving at our awkward adolescent phase—we think we know it all when, in reality, we are suffering from the ignorance of not knowing what we don't know. Psychedelics in the real world are even more complicated than in the clinical one. There are greater risks of careless, uninformed use; unethical practitioners; and self-anointed "shamans" behaving badly.

As a result, local governments have been quicker to pick up the slack, devising new regulations and psychedelic programs that the Feds won't yet touch. There are newly launched regulated psilocybin programs in Oregon and

Colorado, pilot programs for MDMA and psilocybin in hospitals in Utah, and state-funded psilocybin research in Indiana to benefit veterans and first responders. On the ballot in 2024 in Massachusetts was a proposal to decriminalize, in a therapeutic and regulated setting, the growing, consuming, and sharing—no selling—of five different psychedelics including ibogaine, which could make a huge difference for opioid addicts. It didn't pass. Not even close. There's been another new development since this momentous election: Many counties (nearly every one) in Oregon have opted out of their psilocybin programs. We are facing setbacks left and right, but don't let them get you down. There are many who believe in this cause, and I would argue that, at its heart, psychedelic healing is a bipartisan issue. The Department of Veterans Affairs, running the nation's largest health care delivery system, may well pick up the ball and run with it. And the laws are changing every two years, state by state.

What we need now is more education. As the research and legislation evolve, books like this one will help usher us all into a psychedelic adulthood, one where we are forewarned and forearmed with education, and more skilled at making responsible decisions for our spiritual growth.

Oh, the things you'll learn, but painlessly! In *Modern Psychedelics*, Joe guides you through brain science, drug science, and social science. You'll range from a "businessman's trip" on DMT to the real businessmen of the psychedelic venture capital space. Do you need to discern kava from kratom from kanna? I would argue that this is crucial information for conversation in today's polite society. What about the subtleties of DMT and 5-MeO-DMT, or the sexiness of 2-CB versus MDMA, or knowing how to mitigate some of the nausea from eating your magic mushrooms? Again, yes. And beyond learning the differences between LSD, ibogaine, ayahuasca, and mescaline, you may be able to save lives with purity- and potency-testing recommendations and a working knowledge of emergency psychedelic first aid.

The faster you're moving, the farther ahead you need to look.

In these breathless days, there are tools to help us see what's coming and teachers to help us use those tools safely. Venture forth, but be sure you have a good guide. As Joe says, "The better you prepare, the better your chances for a positive experience."

Take your map and compass, your food and water, don't forget the sunscreen, and, of course, pack your well-worn copy of this book.

Godspeed, my friends. Safe travels.

*Julie Holland, MD*
Cape Cod, November 2024

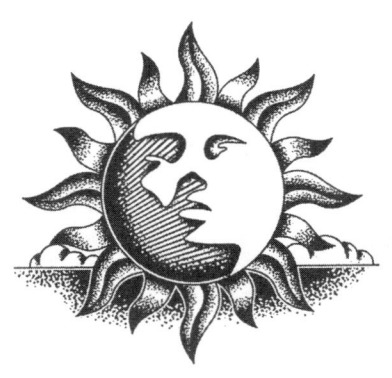

# Author's Note

I t's often recommended that you enlist a guide when embarking on a psychedelic journey. As your guide through this book, allow me to introduce myself.

I'm a former journalist and editor who now makes my living as a communications and executive development coach. I teach people how to speak in public, spread their great ideas to large audiences, and lead their teams more harmoniously (without psychedelics thus far, though I can envision how they might be deployed to increase effectiveness in the future). It's great work that keeps my mind ticking, and I'm privileged to practice it. I am not a scientist, but I understand science and have a knack for getting researchers who speak and write in unfathomably technical ways to explain things simply and clearly. That's my skill. I translate the arcane and complex language of science into words and concepts that people can understand.

I'm generally a happy person, but I suffered a two-year depression in my early fifties. I took the SSRI Lexapro, which lifted me out of despair, but it also squashed my libido and flattened the bright colors in the world into gray tones. Still, unlike half of the population who feel no positive effects from SSRIs, they helped me find beautiful moments that eventually led to beautiful days.

As for psychedelics—I am not the world's most experienced user, nor do I aspire to be. In fact, meditation, which I've practiced fitfully for thirty years, is my preferred medicine. Psychedelics are an occasional, enriching adjunct to life, not its guiding purpose. As is the case for many people, my use has ebbed and flowed with the seasons of my life.

I dabbled with LSD and MDMA as an undergraduate at Northwestern University. (Chicago was one of the distribution hubs of MDMA in the 1970s and 1980s.) Until MDMA was outlawed in 1985, therapists were using it with impressive results. The general consensus was that it made people less afraid of confronting fears, which enabled more open communication with themselves and with others.

MDMA and I became instant great friends. For me, it was gentler than other psychedelics and didn't cause ego dissolution; for this reason, it allowed for more presence of mind. On one MDMA-fueled excursion to the Art Institute of Chicago, I formed a brief, but deep, emotional attachment to Claude Monet's *Water Lilies*. On what felt like a molecular level, I understood the vision underlying this masterpiece (I was never previously moved by impressionism, but on that day, I *loved* it). In college, I had no bad trips, though that wasn't true for everyone in my circle. Psychedelics opened a window into the landscapes of my mind, but in retrospect, I wish I had known more about what they were capable of because my experiences might have been all the richer. Unlike people who relegate their psychedelic explorations to youthful folly, mine have grown more resplendent with age.

I entered adulthood during the War on Drugs and the DARE program, so in the 1980s I quit tripping, fearing that continued use would sizzle my brain—just as they sizzled that egg in the infamous thirty-second "this is your brain on drugs" television spot. (*Side note*: The American Egg Board took issue with that ad, saying that young kids would misconstrue the message and think eggs were harmful. C'mon, Egg Board, kids aren't that dumb!)

My reacquaintance with psychedelics occurred several years ago after I wrote *Brave New Weed*, an investigation into the science and sociology of cannabis, a plant that has been used medicinally for four thousand years and was also grossly maligned by prohibition. I learned then that our brains produce endocannabinoids, which can be loosely described as endogenous versions of THC and CBD. No one knows quite why, but our own brains are factories of illegal drugs! Clearly, there is more to these substances than meets the eye.

There was another factor driving my curiosity, one that members of my generation will understand. By my mid-fifties, I knew that I had to take steps to actively avoid becoming an ossified old man. Even though inwardly I still feel like I'm forty-two, I've seen firsthand that, along with a rigidity of joints and bones, age can too easily bring with it a rigidity of thinking. Habits make life easier—less thinking equals fewer decisions to make. I see it in myself and with friends who are growing disinterested in learning new things or are growing

# "A self that goes on changing is a self that goes on living."

—VIRGINIA WOOLF

cynical and dismissive about the wonders of life. This can leave them feeling left behind or isolated from culture and society, or worse, bitter. Maintaining a flexible mind, tapping into some of that childlike awe, felt paramount to staying vital—even as my body continues its inevitable decline. Having been through years of fifty-minute talk therapy hours and any number of fitness regimes and healthy diets, I had reached the limit of what they could offer. I wanted a deeper jolt, something to make me slightly uncomfortable with my own, privileged status quo. It's an urge adjacent to the urge to travel. Being in a place that's unfamiliar and uncomfortable forces you to see the world with fresh eyes. You may lose your footing, but you learn something about the world and, if you're lucky, about yourself.

Part of my anti-ossification plan came in a heart-shaped chocolate infused with 5 grams of magic mushrooms. That heroic dose, and the subsequent hours of giddy laughter and travels through the contours of my mind, shifted something inside of me that's not easily captured in words. Psychedelics defy conceptual thinking, and mushrooms enabled me to see beyond myself and hold my problems and concerns more lightly. At the time, I knew nothing about what's commonly (and often incorrectly) called neuroplasticity, but that fungus sprouted a slew of new perceptual and neural connections that gently altered the course of my life.

My next experience occurred a year later when a friend invited me to an ayahuasca ceremony in upstate New York. (Once I started to speak openly about my newfound psychedelic path, I seemed to magnetically attract others stumbling forward in a similar direction.)

Two dozen people were spaced out like numbers on a clock around the perimeter of a large yurt on a snowy winter evening. I drank the bittersweet liquor of boiled leaves and bark and waited for the infamous purge that promised to unleash encounters with spirit images. But it never happened. Instead, I endured six hours (it felt like six days) of whiz-bang auditory distortions and visual hallucinations that were more geometric and industrial than inspirational. They were interesting, but emotionally cold. At four in the morning, I visited the bathroom where the purge occurred exuberantly from the other end. It was as if I had let go of something greater than the prior day's meal, the final event of the evening's physical thrashing.

I woke up the next morning feeling mushy and flooded with memories that hadn't visited me in years. In the sharing circle that followed the journey, the ayahuasquero advised me to dive into those feelings of vulnerability. I nodded in silent agreement but had no idea what he was talking about. In the next weeks, I noticed subtle and, at first glance, unremarkable changes. I wasn't craving my regular two cups of morning coffee, and my taste for wine had all but vanished. But when a remastered edition of Bach's cello suites brought me to tears, I understood that the medicine had softened me in an unexpected way. And here we are today . . .

## A Few More Practical Things . . .

This book does not offer medical advice, nor does it recommend that you try psychedelics. In fact, if you encounter anyone who tells you that you *absolutely positively definitely* must take psychedelics, run the other way. Whether to use them is a conversation you should have with yourself, a trusted health practitioner, a mentor, or a spiritual guide. Good guidance is one of the best insurance policies you can obtain.

Just as dosing guidelines on cannabis products have changed the game—users now know that a 5 mg THC gummy is a gentle enhancement, while 100 mg can knock an inexperienced user flat—dosing is key to skilled psychedelic use. The recommendations found under "The Substances" are not infallible—everyone's metabolism and mental condition are different—but they are a good starting point if you're looking to experiment with different magnitudes of journeys. That chapter also outlines the duration of effects, adverse reactions, and drug-drug interactions—all things that skilled users should bear in mind.

Even if you are armed with knowledge, psychedelics can be tricky. It's wise to approach them with respect or, as Terence McKenna counseled, fear. They can take you places you can't imagine. James Fadiman, the author of *The Psychedelic Explorer's Guide* and *Microdosing for Health, Healing, and Enhanced Performance*, who has researched psychedelics since the 1960s (but no longer indulges), echoes McKenna's warning. "When someone says, 'I want to take LSD *but* . . .' I tell them to steer clear until they understand the full depth of their objection." Both men are OGs of psychedelic exploration. Heed their advice.

Along the same lines, beware of what health care professionals are now calling the Pollan

Effect. Michael Pollan's bestselling book *How to Change Your Mind* so effectively made the case for psychedelics that he is now being held responsible for the sky-high expectations people bring to the experience. That's a testament to his estimable narrative skills, but no substance is a direct route to "fixing" your problems or finding yourself. Just like Alice, you will have to tumble down many rabbit holes to find your own Wonderland or whatever it is you're searching for. Science itself is also wandering down a lot of rabbit holes as it struggles to understand psychedelics. Having researched this book, I'm now convinced that wandering seems to me an essential and undervalued part of any quest worth taking.

Another ingredient to wise use: Is your substance itself safe? Psychedelics are not physically harmful (the exception is ibogaine, which at high doses appears to exacerbate arrhythmia), but if they're tainted with chemicals such as fentanyl, or in some cases taken in combination with certain other chemicals, they can kill you. Harm reduction is an inconvenient but necessary conversation today. Chapter 7 introduces you to valuable resources, among them: new-to-market QTests, which determine potency, and the Fireside Project, a hotline service that provides someone to talk to, no matter where in the world, or where in your journey, you happen to be.

And finally, listen to your own voice. If you've decided psychedelics are not for you, follow the advice of the philosopher and writer Alan Watts: "Once you get the message, hang up the phone." On the other hand, if, like ethnopharmacologist Dennis McKenna, you've attended five hundred ayahuasca ceremonies and are still learning, heed the call of the 501st.

## Final Words of Caution

While most people who use psychedelics report positive experiences, using them is not without psychological risks.

It's unwise to try high-dose psychedelics—especially on your own—if you're schizophrenic, bipolar, highly anxious, plagued by emotional trauma, or have any serious psychiatric conditions. People who are vulnerable to psychotic processes or who have a family history of them are at increased risk, particularly if they are in their late teens or early twenties.

Research shows that among people who've used magic mushrooms:

- 11 percent report putting themselves at risk or in risky situations.
- 3 percent sought medical help.
- 10 percent reported adverse psychological symptoms that lasted over a year; 8 percent of those who reported adverse reactions sought treatment.[1]

A year is too long to suffer from unhappiness, especially self-inflicted unhappiness. Another small subset of users attributed the onset of psychosis to having used psychedelics in their youth. That's a lifelong nightmare from which there is no recovery. Chapter 7 discusses some of the underreported psychological and spiritual emergencies that can and will most certainly occur more frequently if and when prohibition is lifted.

## SKILLED USE IS CAUTIOUS USE

There will be casualties in the psychedelic renaissance. We're already seeing a parade of dodgy gurus, cults, and false messiahs; transgressions will occur, and people will get hurt. But you can arm yourself and find ways to be more supported. Use this book as a support.

A small percentage of people become terrified or engage in dangerous behavior while tripping. The probability is low, but it exists. Don't trip in public where you can stumble into others or into traffic, and never trip with people you don't trust.

I refer to challenging trips in this book, but in all honesty the word *challenging* is about as descriptive as calling a climb to Mount Everest *hard*. A challenge can include big emotions such as grief, anguish, sadness, or despair. It can be a frenetic encounter with weirdness or trauma, confrontations with family dynamics, painful insights, or downright scary imagery. A challenge can also be something you learn from.

No two people respond the same way to any substance. I once tripped with a group where we all took 3.5 grams of Penis Envy (PE) mushrooms. One man spent the day in bed, nauseated.

Another woman felt nothing. Someone else danced among the trees for four hours. The rest of us lay on a beach, went swimming, and giggled away the day.

In most places, psychedelics, with the exception of ketamine, are illegal. This is changing, but if breaking the law makes you anxious, skip it. Why subject yourself to the stress?

Ram Dass once said, "For grass you should have the equivalent of a driver's license. And for LSD you should have the equivalent of a pilot's license."[2]

This book won't provide the license, but it will offer you some help in getting the plane off the ground, into the right flight path, and safely landed. It will help you reduce unexpected turbulence and alert you if you shouldn't be flying at all. The best way to ensure a good journey is to be informed, because here, at the beginning of the psychedelic resurgence, curiosity is outpacing laws, sensible regulation, and best practices.

So be smart. Prepare for your experience. Understand your intent. Have a mind-blowing or—as research seems to be indicating—a mind-growing time!

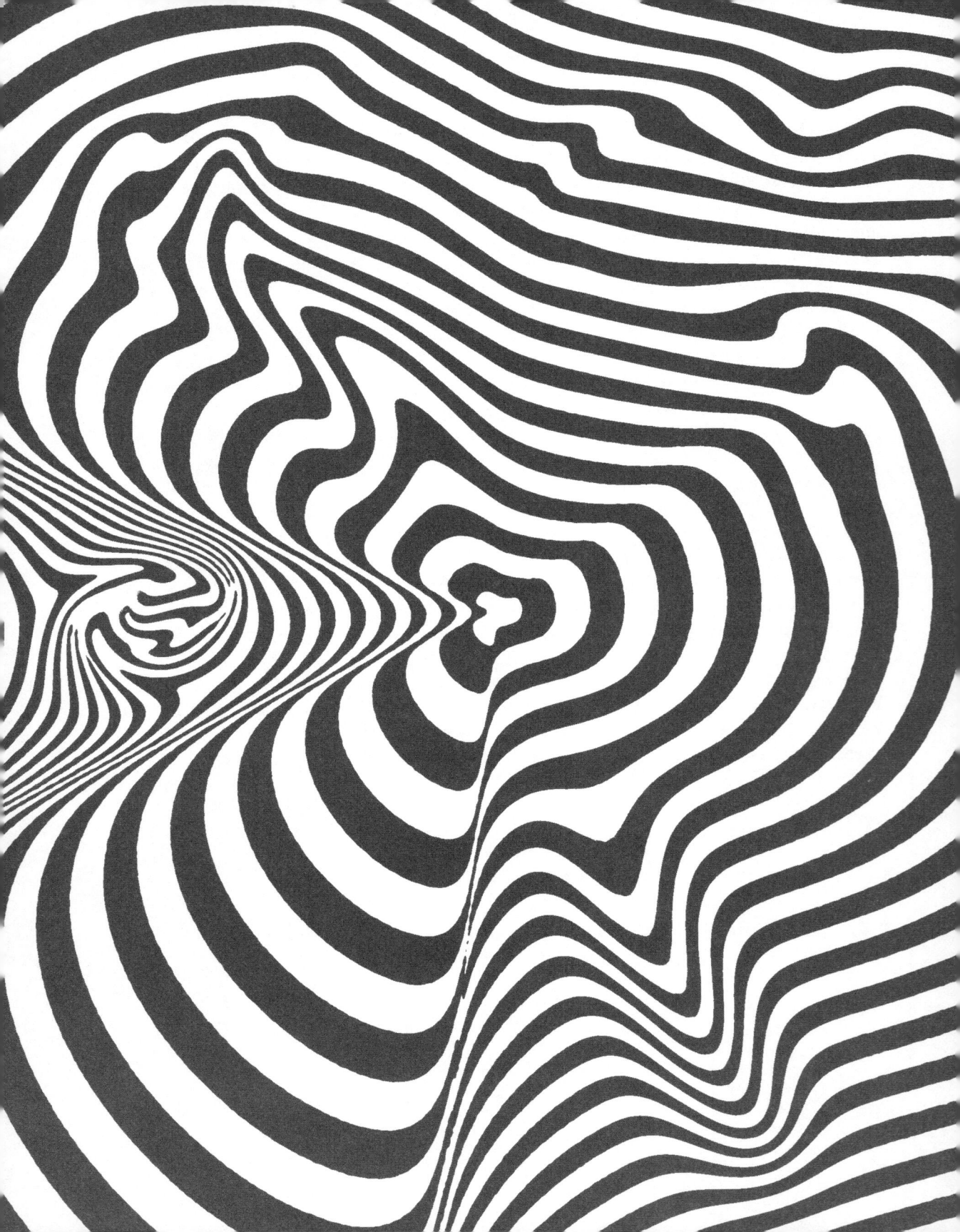

# CHAPTER 1

# WELCOME TO THE PSYCHEDELIC RESURGENCE

------------------------------------------------------------

*The way we see the world shapes the way we treat it. If a mountain is a deity, not a pile of ore . . . if a forest is a sacred grove, not timber; if other species are biological kin, not resources; or if the planet is our mother, not an opportunity— then we will treat each other with greater respect. This is the challenge, to look at the world from a different perspective.*

DAVID SUZUKI, *Canadian geneticist and environmental activist*

The following conversations occurred over two days in 2023. I did not initiate these conversations, and there isn't one word of writerly embellishment in these accounts.

- A psychologist acquaintance tells me he's going away for two weeks to Mexico. I love Mexico, so I ask him where he's heading. To an ibogaine clinic to help him kick a substance abuse problem he has grappled with for years, he tells me. He's excited but nervous because one ibogaine trip can last for a grueling thirty-six hours.
- A publisher exec I know is away for a weekend ayahuasca ceremony in the hope of getting a new perspective on her working life. She has arrhythmia and is wondering if two ceremonies back-to-back will strain her heart.* What have I heard?
- Two months ago, my friend JJ found Joyous, a service that mails a two-month supply of low-dose ketamine lozenges to his home. "A life changer," he told me. After sixty days and a few Zoom check-ins with a doctor, he's finally beating a lifelong struggle with depression. He wants to know if the happy effects will disappear if he stops.**
- Robert, a retired communications executive in the nonprofit sector, joined the

---

\* DMT, a key ingredient in ayahuasca, can raise the heart rate.

\*\* It's not definitively known how long the antidepressant effects of ketamine last, but indications are that treatments have to be continued. Ketamine does enable plasticity in the brain, but the window of plasticity is thought to be the shortest of all psychedelics—about four days.

Zide Door Church in West Oakland, California. The church legally dispenses entheogenic plants (magic mushrooms and cannabis) to "parishioners." He bought 7 grams of mushrooms ($60) and calls to ask how much he should take and if I know any hack to avoid getting nauseous.

· A neurodivergent colleague read in an online forum that LSD helps people break free of the behaviors that emotionally cage them in. I have no knowledge, but I sent him Aaron Paul Orsini's book, *Autism on Acid*.*

· A client confides that he read my book *Brave New Weed: Adventures into the Uncharted World of Cannabis*, and that he's been microdosing with psilocybin for five months. (Apparently *Brave New Weed* is a gateway book—people presume, not unreasonably, that I know a lot about every substance because I know a lot about cannabis.) He wants to switch to LSD because dosing is easier and more consistent than with the many varieties of fungi that grow in the ground. Do I have a source?**

· I was struggling with the lingering effects of COVID for three weeks—lightheaded, exhausted, and foggy brained. I shared my woes with my LSD microdosing buddy—we began together three years ago—and he fired back, "It's not COVID, dude. It's withdrawal! You stopped cold turkey two months ago when you went to Mexico.

LSD takes weeks to clear the system." I scoured half a dozen papers, books, and online forums on the topic but not one mentioned "withdrawal." Most forums say that LSD clears the brain/body in three days, but there's no definitive research about microdosing. Some claim the benefits I feel are the result of expectancy effects. I'm okay with that.

It's an exciting and confusing time in the world of psychedelics. There's a lot of hope and an increasing amount of hype about these substances. Drugs that twenty years ago were said to sizzle the brain or make you crazy are now being used to make you saner. The US Controlled Substances Act still outlaws psychedelics as Schedule 1 "narcotics" that have "no medical value and have a high rate of addiction." Although Phase III clinical trials for MDMA to treat post-traumatic stress disorder (PTSD) concluded with promising results, and despite the fact that the country of Australia has legalized MDMA-assisted therapy to treat PTSD,*** the US Food and Drug Administration has—frustratingly and sadly for the thirteen million Americans suffering from the condition—refused to approve its use in the States. This has dampened some of the effervescent optimism, but the correction has also attuned the public to the hype and made people more aware of risks as accessibility to these substances increases. This is a good thing as it paints a more realistic safety profile for all users.

---

* In *Autism on Acid: How LSD Helped Me Understand, Navigate, Alter and Appreciate My Autistic Perceptions*, neurodivergent author Orsini cites research that LSD appears to ease the social anxiety that accompanies autism.

** My source, a chemist, doesn't accept referrals.

*** As of this writing, regulatory issues have restricted the number of therapists approved to prescribe MDMA to a few dozen.

Of course, people aren't waiting for legal or scientific permission to try psychedelics. One 2010 study[1] estimated that thirty-two million Americans called themselves lifetime psychedelic users. There's no way to know how many millions more there are today, but stellar books like Michael Pollan's *How to Change Your Mind* and Ayalet Waldman's *A Really Good Day*, as well as films like *Fantastic Fungi*, have pushed these compounds out of the shadows and into the spotlight. Psychedelics are at a tipping point (or "tripping point?") of acceptance.

The excitement is apparent in popular culture as well as the more sober reaches of science. Not long ago, psychedelics were career killers in scientific research; they were only whispered about in back offices. Today, if chemists and neuroscientists don't mention them, it's to protect the patents they've applied for. August institutions—Yale, Harvard, Berkeley, New York University, and Johns Hopkins among them—have established research centers that are turning out studies showing that psychedelics when combined with therapy can effectively treat depression, PTSD, end-of-life anxiety, and a host of stubborn illnesses that elude modern medicine. Not uncommonly, one or two treatments offer relief that endures for months, sometimes years. That's an entirely different paradigm from the one-pill-a-day-for-the-rest-of-your-life solutions currently offered by psychiatry.

The boom isn't only happening in academia. Institutes are popping up across the world to train guides and therapists, and at the moment, demand far exceeds supply.* While a host of early-to-market companies have fizzled, the surviving biopharma start-ups are racing to synthesize next-generation "pseudodelics" that deliver therapeutic results without the "side effects" of the trip. Psychedelic advocates view this as an apostate attempt to medicalize the magic of these compounds—the trip is where the revelations occur!—and a robust movement has sprung up to counter such pursuits. In June 2023, the Psychedelic Science conference sponsored by the Multidisciplinary Association for Psychedelic Studies (MAPS) drew twelve thousand participants—four times the size of its conference three years before and the same number of attendees as the American Psychiatric Association's meeting. Melissa Etheridge, Jaden Smith, and conservative Republican governor Rick Perry (!) were among the star speakers.

Remember how people once asked, "What's your sign?" The opening question at MAPS was, "What's your medicine?"

As word spreads, access is expanding. If you're depressed and the ketamine-in-a-box method mentioned above makes you nervous, pop into a center in a growing number of cities for an IV or nasal infusion. Companies like Nushama administer ketamine in a comfortable yet clinical setting at a steeper price than home delivery—$400 to $850 a session compared with $200 a month. A more sensual therapeutic experience is offered by Cardea, a ketamine-assisted wellness and treatment clinic in New York City, where every element of the decor, from window shutters to lamps and tables, is constructed from sheets of dried mushroom mycelium—an interior design truly befitting the word *trippy*. After an hour of intention setting, you'll be tucked into a cozy, fabric-draped, iron-frame bed. The medicine sends you into space while a therapist

---

* One example: The UC Berkeley Center for the Science of Psychedelics offers a $10,000 Facilitation Certificate Program that includes two hundred hours of instruction, weekend immersions, online learning, contemplative practice, and a five-day psilocybin retreat.

guides your journey with a live sound bath of singing bells and gongs to melt your normal beta brain waves to a more relaxed alpha frequency and potentiate the healing effects of ketamine. It worked for me!

If you're eyeing a retreat, you might head to a center in Jamaica, where you'll trip on psilocybin Monday, Wednesday, and Friday, and do art or music integration on the off days . . . or maybe you'd prefer Tandava, the world's first 5-MeO-DMT wellness center in the village of Tepoztlán, Mexico's newly minted center for healing. There are psilocybin retreats for couples in the Catskills or so-called Medicine Women's Retreats for women over fifty. The Jungle Gayborhood in Costa Rica gathers queer men to "consciously explore embodiment practices, sacred plant ceremonies, permaculture, and sacred sexuality." For a more indigenous ayahuasca experience, consider flying to the Peruvian Amazon, where you might live in a hut, eat the traditional restricted *dieta*, eliminate all sexual activities including with yourself, and attend ceremonies led by a native shaman, or in some unfortunate cases by a native huckster parading as a shaman. The rush of tourists to the Amazon has sparked protests by environmental groups concerned that the rising tide of cultural appropriation and so-called extractive capitalism is threatening the limited supply of visionary plants and the indigenous ways of life.

If you'd rather exercise your green thumb, there is no shortage of inexpensive instructional courses (or free YouTube videos) on home cultivation of magic mushrooms. It's legal! Home cultivation too messy? Scroll through Instagram to locate a service that will deliver mushrooms to your home or office.

There's a deluge of information swirling around the internet—some of it good, lots of it suspect, most of it marketing—but there are still so many unknowns. As the shackles on the almost sixty-year-old prohibition loosen and curiosity skyrockets, there's one thing missing: a judgment-free handbook that draws together contemporary science, ancient wisdom, and best practices to guide people in using these powerful substances to their maximum benefit and to avoid preventable problems. I suspect you agree, since you're holding such a book in your hand.

## Mindful Use Is Smart Use

What exactly is mindful use of psychedelics? I believe it begins with education. Education about what psychedelics are (and are not), what they can do (and cannot), who should use them (and who should not), and what elements of a trip you can control (and how to best prepare for what you can't). It's knowing how to dose, what to expect, and how to arrange your external and internal conditions to maximize benefits, mitigate risks, and make meaning from the jumble of images, thoughts, visions, and mystical/magical moments that will occur.[*]

Having a trusted guide is another key to ensuring the best outcome. Consider this book one of your trusted guides.

As the author of *Brave New Weed*, which sought to set the record straight on cannabis, I have spent many hours speaking to advocates and foes of substances. I can assure you that the two groups are equally strident in

---

[*] It's also knowing that eating a healthy diet, getting good sleep, staying hydrated, and choosing not to combine substances wantonly are essential elements to all drug experimentation.

their positions. But skilled use is not binary; it's neither all pro nor all con. It's understanding that there is a middle ground that can be safely navigated.

So before digging in, let's get a few things straight.

1. **Psychedelics are drugs, but they don't act like pharmaceuticals.**

   The term *pharmaceutical* generally refers to a compound that acts the same way each time it is administered. This is not the case with psychedelics. Even when dosing is consistent, the effects are predictably unpredictable. Albert Hofmann, the father of LSD, said, "In spite of a good mood at the beginning of a session—positive expectations,beautiful surroundings, and sympathetic company—I once fell into a terrible depression. The unpredictability of effects is the major danger of LSD."[2] The same is true for every substance in this book.

   Also, the category of psychedelics has expanded from the so-called classic psychedelics: LSD, psilocybin, DMT/5-MeO-DMT, ayahuasca, peyote/mescaline. MDMA is classified as an empathogen or entactogen. Ketamine is a dissociative anesthetic. Ibogaine is an oneirogen, something capable of iducing a dream state. Classifications aside, all of these substances work by changing the perception of reality and the circuitry in the brain.

2. **Psychedelics have been misunderstood for centuries.**

   Although they have been used on every continent since long before history was recorded, psychedelics are disruptors. They are understood by the people who use them but feared by the powers that want to control them. That fear is not unwarranted. Traditionally, psychedelics have been administered in group settings led by a curandero, shaman, or healer. He (and it is more often than not a "he") is responsible for dosing and watching over the proceedings. He chooses who gets which substances and how much, and ensures that the participants understand the rules of engagement. Rather than upsetting the social order, psychedelics are used to preserve it. When a young Huichol is initiated into manhood, drinking peyote allows him to know for himself the spirit world that rules the entire tribe's worldview. The Huichol don't use laws to control "drug use"; their rituals control it.

   When psychedelics were unleashed in the 1960s with no one in charge, a form of societal chaos ensued. In their panic, the authorities clamped down, imposing draconian laws and halting research into what were, at the time, considered promising medicines.

3. **Psychedelics don't impose anything on our minds; rather they amplify access to what is already there.**

   The word *psychedelic* comes from the Greek *psyche*—mind—and *delic*, which means "manifesting." Dr. Stanislav Grof, a pioneer of psychedelic therapy who administered over four thousand trips, called psychedelics "nonspecific amplifiers" of thoughts, emotions, and perceptions. Grief that you may not have fully metabolized may surface. You might hear colors, or you might be walking through a meadow and suddenly *understand* the sound of a bird in a way that makes you cry.

4. **Most psychedelics are not physically harmful or addictive.**

Unlike opiates, alcohol, cocaine, or tobacco, psychedelics taken on their own and in proper doses will not kill you or cause dependence. (Ketamine excepted—it can be habit forming when used off-label.) Nor do they typically create drug-seeking behavior. The probability of getting baboons to self-administer cocaine in lab experiments is 100 percent. This is not the case with psychedelics, because unlike cocaine they don't directly drive the dopamine system. Rather, most psychedelics tend to leave you satisfied and not wanting more for months or years, or in some cases ever. That said, certain psychedelics do have drug-drug interactions that can put people with heart or psychiatric conditions at risk.

5. **Psychedelics are not an escape from reality.**

Plumbing the depths of your psyche to get to an insight usually requires work, and what is revealed is not always beautiful or pleasant. The insight may come instantly or it may unfold over time. Nor do psychedelics make returning to "ordinary" life more difficult. They can, however, make ordinary life less ordinary.

If you're trying to escape reality, it's wiser to try to change that reality than run away from it.

6. **Psychedelics are medicines, but wholly distinct from other medicines we know.**

Modern medicines target specific disease states, but psychedelics display a category-busting cross-diagnostic efficacy. In addition to depression, PTSD, and cluster headaches, they are now being tested to counter opioid, alcohol, and tobacco addiction; the pain caused by fibromyalgia; early Alzheimer's; OCD; stuttering; Parkinson's disease; the lingering effects of Lyme disease; and anorexia, which has recently been identified as the deadliest mental illness. Preliminary results across the board are promising.

7. **Psychedelics enable new connections in the mind, in the brain, and between people.**

Each substance causes a distinct set of subjective feelings. LSD, for example, is said to be pushier and more insistent—a bit bitchier—than the warmer, gentler, and generally uplifting state brought on by magic mushrooms. The effects of mescaline are described as more numinous than those of a reality-shattering blast of 5-MeO-DMT. But all these substances create neuronal and synaptic connections in the brain that can, under the right conditions, enable new learning and healing—even in older brains. How we take advantage of these openings is up to us.

8. **Psychedelics don't only treat illnesses.**

Most clinical research focuses on medical conditions—no institution is going to fund a study on increasing awe or fun. But psychedelics can be used to access more of your human potential. They can help you circumvent a creative rut or break free of habits that no longer serve you. MDMA can help couples connect and care for each other or fight in more compassionate ways. This has been known since the 1970s.

9. **Psychedelics can enable feelings of oneness with humanity and the natural world.**

Psychedelics enable a unity consciousness with animals, plants, trees, and other beings. Experiments from the 1960s that were followed up in the 1980s, and replicated again under stricter research conditions in 2006, showed that psilocybin sparked mystical or spiritual awakenings that subjects rated among the top five most important experiences of their lives—not just a fun memory from a party weekend, but something as resonant as the birth of a child or death of a parent. The late Roland Griffiths, the founding director of the Johns Hopkins Center for Psychedelic and Consciousness Research, believed that these feelings of connection could "provide the basis for moral and ethical principles that would lessen the likelihood that humanity will drive itself off a cliff."

Whether or not psychedelics can stave off Armageddon, it's important to know that Griffiths was no wishful dreamer. He was a strict evidence-based psychopharmacologist and drug abuse specialist who over five decades published 402 papers and was cited almost forty thousand times. He was the first to study the effects of psilocybin therapy on people with end-of-life anxiety; his 2006 study on mystical experience and the alleviation of depression got the research ball rolling. His thoughtful opinions were based on rigorous clinical investigations. He's worth paying attention to.

10. **Psychedelics can be great fun.**

Aldous Huxley called a psychedelic trip a "holiday from the self," a busting-out from our own small egos. (In the still-Puritan culture of the US, *joy* may be a more acceptable word than *fun*.) While some people don't think fun is the highest order or best use of these substances, I respectfully disagree. I have used MDMA and LSD at raves and festivals and experienced an emotional openness and collective effervescence with everyone around me—I've often suspected that the social and relational aspects of the experience, not the drug, are the real medicine. These celebrations are also among the few non-religious rituals available in our data-driven, hyper-individualized, screen-based culture. At average doses, they also enable laughter and fellowship, not to mention jubilation, glee, delight, and exuberance, all excellent ingredients for well-being, especially since they place no burden on anyone else.

The better you prepare, the better your chances for a positive experience. Thoughtfully honing your intentions, choosing the company you're with, creating a comfortable setting, and knowing where not to go when high are key ingredients to safer, wiser use. Chapter 4 offers practical and imaginative ways to better set yourself up for success.

11. **Psychedelics lift the hood on consciousness.**

Even if psychedelics can't provide answers, they do provide clues that, under the right guidance, can be revelatory of the way our minds work. This causes me, and many others, to wonder if there isn't a larger reason why these magic plants and molecules were put on earth.

# "Hallucinogens are the shamanic medicine par excellence, but now they're finding their way almost magically, almost shamanically, into very traditional halls of Western medicine."

—MARK PLOTKIN, ethnobotanist, conservationist, and president of the Amazon Conservation Team

12. **Psychedelics are not the only way to explore the workings of your mind or heart.**

While headlines froth over psychedelics as the latest, greatest quick fixes to everything that ails us, meditation, yoga, prayer, music, journaling, art, and psychotherapy also offer insights into the mind and psyche. There are many commonalities among these internal, reflective practices and psychedelics. I look forward to the lifting of prohibition so those intersections can be more fully understood. Until then, we will continue to explore on our own or with our communities.

## WILL PSYCHEDELICS MAKE ME FAIL A DRUG TEST?

If your work subjects you to drug testing and you feel anxious about it, don't risk taking any substance. However, bear in mind that the current standard ten-panel drug test detects marijuana, amphetamines, opioids, barbiturates, PCP, methadone, methaqualone, and propoxyphene but not psychedelics. *Please note:* MDMA (which is confusingly classified as an amphetamine but does not contain the drug amphetamine) will show up on a standard urine test up to seventy-two hours after use. The ten-panel test does not look for any other substances covered in this book, but for your information, here is a list of detection windows for urine tests:

- MDMA—72 hours
- Ketamine—14 to 30 days, depending on quantity used
- LSD/DMT/psilocybin/mescaline— 1 day, super hard to test for, almost never done
- Marijuana—1 to 30 days

## A Word about Sources

Where possible, I have included the findings of clinical trials in all discussions. I understand the irony that clinical trials, which are based on defining and constraining variables, are the least psychedelic way of exploring these mind-expanding compounds, but science and measurement are the best tools we have to distinguish fact from fiction.

Beyond fMRI scans and clinical protocols, though, it would be impudent to ignore what millions of users have reported about psychedelics over the decades. The thousands of "citizen scientists" in Reddit forums, or who have joined the Microdose.me study, also have insights worth noting, especially because there are few sources of funding to study illegal substances for the purposes of "increasing motivation," "augmenting sexual pleasure," or "feeling more focused" even if scientists were able to measure such states. Some of the common hacks that people are using every day are covered in this book.

And crucially, the wisdom accumulated by indigenous peoples over thousands of years must have a place in this book and in all conversations about psychedelics going forward. No one knows how our ancestors learned to prepare decoctions from visionary plants or what led them to create ceremonies that support transformational healing. Shamans like to say the plants gave them the instructions, and as confounding as this is to the Western mind, there's no evidence to the contrary. The practice a mystery that I can't explain but that I humbly accept as another of life's many mysteries, an acceptance based on my own experience and that of wise explorers and esteemed scientists. It's too compelling to dismiss as woo woo.

Clinical trials are the gold standard in Western medicine, but many gold-standard professionals believe different investigative tools are needed to truly understand the workings of these substances. Until those methods are developed, there's a rich body of knowledge within the worldwide community of practitioners and celebrants. This book values and collects wisdom from these sources.

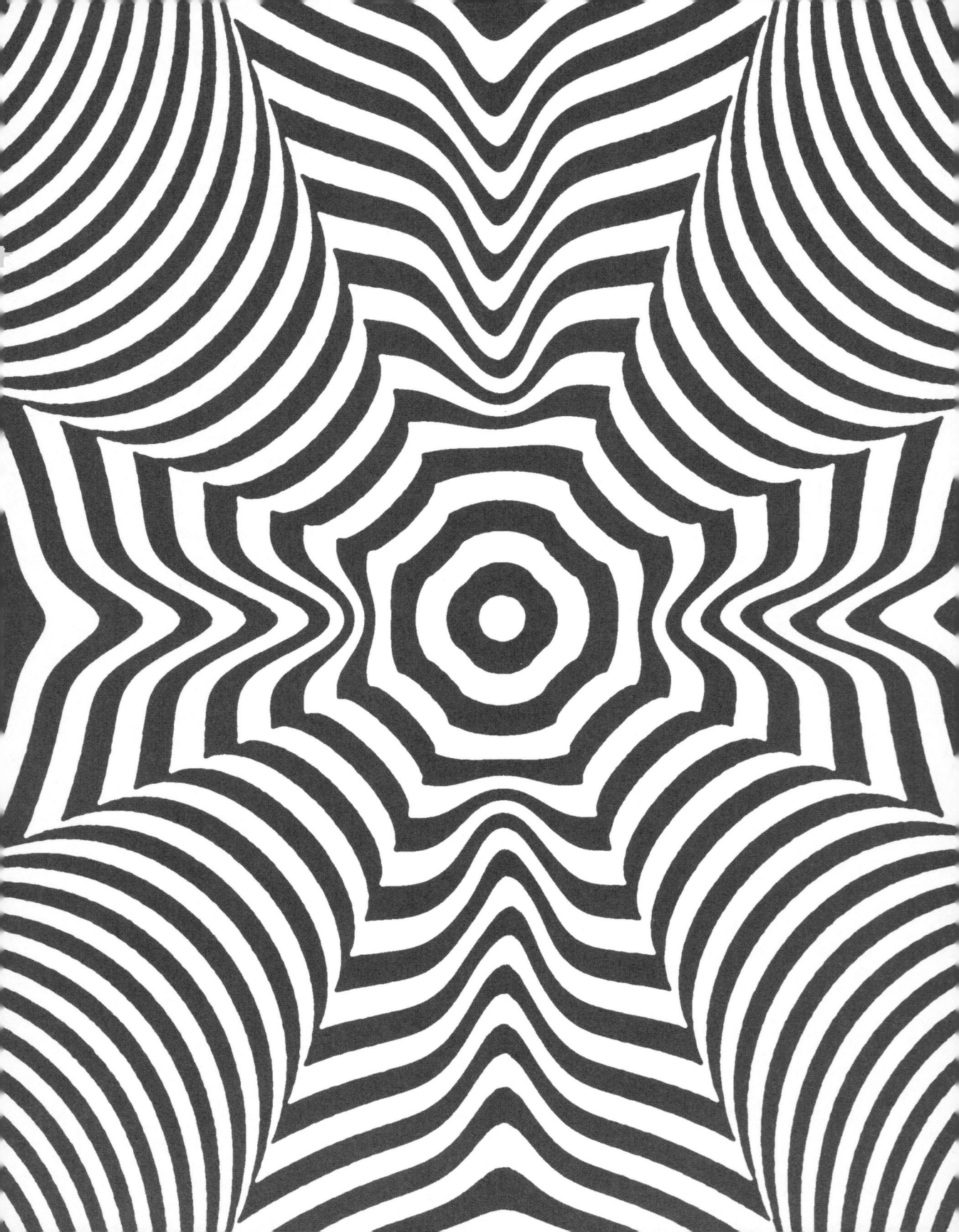

# CHAPTER 2

# BIRTH, BAN, BOOM!

## PSYCHEDELICS IN HISTORY

------------------------------------------

How you gonna keep 'em down on the farm after they've seen Paree?

JAMES FADIMAN, *in answer to the question*
*"How did psychedelics affect the course of your life?"*

W hat follows is a selective and by no means comprehensive account of the long, strange history of psychedelics in the West.

### The First Wave: Birth

Human beings and psychedelics have been on a journey together for far longer than history has been recorded. Whether it's Navajo peyote rituals, Amazonian ayahuasca ceremonies, or 1960s LSD Be-Ins, the pursuit of chemically induced states of heightened consciousness has spanned cultures and has outlived thousands of years of murder, oppression, and prohibition.

The oldest psychedelic artifact, from 6800 BCE to 6200 BCE was a fossilized San Pedro cactus found in the mountains of Peru.[1] There are drawings of mushrooms on vessels found in the deserts of North Africa and in the Siberian

ice fields that date back six thousand years. It is thought that the ancient Greeks brewed ergot, the fungus from which LSD is derived, into wine decoctions that were the central sacrament of a secret, multiday ceremony known as the Eleusinian Mysteries, a ritual that persisted for two thousand years. Plato, Aristotle, and Euripides were among its attendees. The flights of magic mushrooms inspired religious awe and communal healing among Mayan, Aztec, and native North Americans until the conquistadors brutally tried to suppress these rituals to enforce the authority of the Catholic Church. US territorial governors spent a century trying to wipe out peyote—and with it, the tribes that consider it an integral part of their identities. It took decades of court battles for the US to finally legalize the cactus for "religious use" in the 1990s.

Psychedelics made their way into modern Western culture without much ado initially.

**PSYCHEDELIC TIMELINE OF DISCOVERY IN THE WEST**

**6500 BCE**—San Pedro cactus is found in a cave in Peru, the earliest evidence of humans' use of psychedelics.

**2000 BCE**—Ergot is possibly used to make the potion called *kykeon*, part of the Eleusinian Mysteries of ancient Greece.

Ibogaine was extracted from the West African *Tabernanthe iboga* shrub in 1867. It was sold as a "stimulating tonic" in France and Belgium, but colonial Europeans remained ignorant of the central role it played in the cultures of Gabon and Cameroon. The German chemist Arthur Heffter separated mescaline crystals from peyote in 1897. He tested it on himself* and named it mescal, but it failed to spark medicinal or popular interest outside of small artistic circles. MDMA was synthesized by Merck pharmaceuticals in 1912 as a compound to control bleeding; its powerful empathogenic qualities went unrecognized until the 1970s. In fact, the entire class of visionary compounds attracted little interest until a microscopic amount of lysergic acid diethylamide (LSD) grazed the skin of Swiss chemist Albert Hofmann's hand in 1943.

In 1938, as the now familiar story goes, Hofmann was working for Swiss pharmaceutical company Sandoz (now Novartis), synthesizing drugs from the rye fungus ergot. He was hoping to find an analeptic compound that would stimulate the circulatory and respiratory systems.[2] He named the twenty-fifth version of the drug LSD-25, but it proved unsuccessful, so it was shelved and Hofmann moved on to other projects.

Five years later, on the morning of April 16, 1943, the thirty-seven-year-old chemist woke up with a "peculiar presentiment" to resynthesize LSD-25 one more time. When later asked why he returned to that particular molecule, he said, "I did not choose LSD. LSD found and called me."[3]

Ergot derivatives are famously potent, so Hofmann, ever the meticulous Swiss scientist, handled it with extreme caution. Presumably, an infinitesimal trace touched his finger. Within an hour he was feeling pleasantly strange, and so he left his lab. Once home and in bed, he closed his eyes to block the blinding daylight and to watch the dance of "kaleidoscopic, fantastic images . . . alternating, variegated, opening and then closing themselves in circles and spirals, exploding in colored fountains, rearranging and hybridizing themselves in constant flux."[4] It lasted only three hours, but his curiosity was piqued.

Back in his lab the following Monday, Hofmann dissolved what he thought was a minuscule dose—250 micrograms (a microgram is one millionth of a gram)—in water and drank it.* He was certain that such a tiny dose** would have no effect, but within forty minutes he was flying. His vision pulsed, he laughed at nothing in particular, but then he was struck by the "ugliness of the technical world" and the sight of his white-coated colleagues, so he asked his assistant, Susi Ramstein, to escort him home. Because of wartime restrictions on automobiles, they hopped on bicycles. That now famous seven-kilometer ride in which the buttoned-up scientist pedaled furiously

---

* Self-testing was standard practice for scientists of that era.

** It was unknown at the time, but LSD is five thousand to ten thousand times as potent as mescaline.

---

**1500 BCE**—A sophisticated fungus cult exists in Guatemala, as evidenced by archaeological "mushroom stones."

**1560 CE**—Spanish missionary priest Bernardino de Sahagún writes about peyote and teonanacatl mushrooms, used by the Aztecs.

**1851**—English ethnobotanist Richard Spruce observes the Tukano Indians in Brazil drinking a visionary tea made from the ayahuasca vine.

## SUSI RAMSTEIN

Albert Hofmann was the first person to trip on LSD, but his lab assistant, twenty-two-year-old Susi Ramstein, got her boss home and helped him navigate the toughest challenges of his psychedelic journey.

A few months after Hofmann's fateful bicycle ride, Susi took 100 mcg of LSD and hopped a tram home. People's faces, especially their noses, grew to comic proportions, which made her laugh, but her ideas remained clear and she maintained control. She shared her experience with colleagues at Sandoz, and her insights may have contributed to figuring out dosage levels for the medical use of LSD. In total, she had three trips, some of which were with the milder psychoactive variants that Hofmann went on to synthesize.

no human had ever experienced LSD's mind-bending effects. His nice neighbor appeared as a "malevolent, insidious witch," and the world pulsed in vibrant colors. The floor bulged, walls wobbled, "especially strange was how all acoustic perceptions, like the sound of a passing car, were transposed into optical sensations, such that every sound triggered a colorful image."[5] Hofmann insisted Susi call his doctor, who after examining him, pronounced him fine. His trip continued until eleven that evening. The next morning Hofmann awoke refreshed and chipper. "Everything glistened and sparkled in a fresh light . . . All my senses vibrated in a condition of highest sensitivity, which persisted for the entire day."[6]

Hofmann was no stranger to mystical experiences—he had had several as a young boy playing in the forest near his hometown village—and he was certain that LSD was bringing him to similar transcendental heights. Perhaps it could be used to answer some of the hard questions about consciousness, or maybe it could be an important psychiatric medicine. But first the chemists at Sandoz had to figure out what on earth this strange-acting chemical was.*

home with electric visions exploding in his head turned out to be unexpectedly adventurous. April 19 is now celebrated the world over as Bicycle Day.

In his original 1943 recounting, Hofmann was convinced he was dying or going insane—

Almost from its inception, LSD suffered an identity crisis from which it has never fully recovered. Arthur Stoll, president of Sandoz, was certain that low doses could help heal

---

* LSD passed animal safety trials, but the animals had some curious reactions. Hofmann noted that mice showed "alterations in licking behavior." Aquarium fish "swam oddly." Low LSD doses caused spiders to weave webs that were "better proportioned and more exactly built than normally. Higher doses led to shoddy construction."

**1867**—Iboga debuts at the Paris Exposition. Fifty years later, tonics made from iboga plant extracts become popular stimulants in France and Belgium.

**1897**—Chemist Arthur Heffter consumes 150 mg of mescaline hydrochloride, confirming mescaline as the main psychedelic component in peyote.

**1912**—MDMA is first synthesized by Merck pharmaceuticals in Germany.

the trauma of the hundreds of millions of Europeans whose lives had been torn apart by World War II. He constructed a "trip chamber" in the company's headquarters in Basel, Switzerland, outfitted with chairs and chaises where employees could take a small 20 or 30 mcg dose and then report effects to a secretary outside.[7] Results were overwhelmingly positive, but Stoll's idea never took flight. Eventually, in what was surely the world's first crowdsourced drug trial, Sandoz made LSD, renamed Delysid for commercial purposes, available at no cost to psychiatrists and researchers who were interested in experimenting with it on themselves or on patients. It came in two formats—a 25 mcg pill and a 100 mcg ampule. At the time, psychiatry was searching for a biochemical root to psychosis and schizophrenia. Sandoz hoped LSD could serve as a "psychotomimetic," a compound that would mimic the psychotic state and reveal to psychiatrists some hidden clues about the illness.

The notion of "set" and "setting" was years away from being articulated. This meant that LSD was at times administered in pleasant offices with a doctor present; less fortunate patients were given massive doses (800 mcg), strapped to hospital beds, and left alone for many terrifying hours to be observed via two-way mirrors. Unsurprisingly, these uncontrolled experiments yielded wildly different accounts of LSD's effects.

Not only were shrinks enlisted as Sandoz shamans, but spies were, too. In the 1950s, as the Cold War unfolded, the US was convinced, not without reason, that the Soviet Union was weaponizing LSD and other chemicals as brainwashing tools they called incapacitating agents. The CIA, then in just its sixth year of infancy, launched its now infamous MK-Ultra program, which clandestinely tested LSD (and mescaline) on thousands of unwitting US citizens and military personnel without their consent and then subjected them to interrogations. This "psychochemical" part of program, which became the basis of the film *The Manchurian Candidate*, continued until a soldier's suicide shut down the operation.

## WORD GOT OUT

In 1953, Abram Hoffer and Humphry Osmond, two psychiatrists working in Canada, were experimenting with LSD to treat alcohol addiction. Having observed that some alcoholics could quit drinking only after a torturous episode of delirium tremens, the spasms and confusion caused by withdrawal, they began giving high doses of LSD to patients, trying to create a horrible experience that would scare them away from alcohol. To their surprise, patients enjoyed it. "In spite of everything we tried . . . they'd have a good experience," Hoffer reported. "They felt good, they saw strange things, they were excited about it."[8]

> **Psychedelic:** "Mind manifesting"
> **Hallucinogen:** "To wander in the mind"
> **Entheogen:** "God within"

---

**1930**—Over a dozen American states outlaw the use and possession of peyote.

**1931**—DMT is synthesized by British chemist Richard Manske and named nigerine.

**1938**—Albert Hofmann synthesizes LSD-25 for Sandoz in Switzerland.

## PSYCHEDELIC ETYMOLOGY

The relationship between Aldus Huxley and Humphry Osmond gave us the word *psychedelic*. In their correspondence following Huxley's trip, they tried to coin a less medical name than "psychomimetic" that better befitted these extraordinary compounds. After a few nonstarters—phanerothyme was one of them—Osmond finally came up with this rhyme:

*To make this trivial world sublime,*
*Take half a gramme of*
*   phanerothyme.*
*To fathom Hell or go angelic*
*Just take a pinch of psychedelic.*

Those unexpected outcomes forced Osmond and Hoffer to pivot. Rather than scaring alcoholics into sobriety, they took the opposite tack and tried to induce mystical experiences in pleasant "living room" surroundings with eye masks and music, supporting patients if difficulties occurred. This was the first inkling that what occurs inside a person's mind ("set") and the outer environment ("setting") could powerfully influence the outcome of an LSD experience. The revised approach succeeded wildly. Almost half of the subjects quit alcohol and stayed clean for over a year. Bill W., cofounder of Alcoholics Anonymous, came to a similar understanding of LSD's anti-addictive power in 1956 when he sampled it in a VA hospital. Wilson was so impressed, he lobbied AA to integrate LSD into its program, but the board nixed the idea of treating one addiction with another drug. Wilson continued experimenting on his own.[9]

It was now clear that LSD was not mirroring a psychotic state. After many attempts at finding a word that best expressed its shapeshifting powers, Osmond, in a letter to Aldous Huxley, came up with the word *psychedelic* from the Greek—*psyche* meaning "mind" and *delic* meaning "manifesting."

Word of psychedelics' power started to seep into the wider culture when Aldous Huxley, who had been in a state of psychological and spiritual fragility, asked Osmond to give him 400 mg of mescaline. The following year Huxley published *The Doors of Perception*, which rhapsodized the power of this drug and which inspired other writers, William Burroughs and Allen Ginsberg the most famous among them, to pursue psychedelics. The book famously framed the mind as a "reducing valve" that limits the vast ocean of perceptual, emotional, and cognitive inputs into a more limited stream of waking consciousness so that humans can function. Psychedelics, he posited, opened the doors to the expanded reality that is normally closed off.

By the early 1960s, psychiatrists had administered LSD to some forty thousand patients. Over a thousand papers described it as an effective treatment for alcoholism, depression, and end-of-life anxiety in patients with cancer.

**April 16, 1943—**
History's first acid trip.

**April 19, 1943—**Hofmann takes 250 µg of LSD and bicycles home while tripping balls. This day is now celebrated as Bicycle Day.

**1947—**Sandoz markets LSD as a psychiatric drug under the name Delysid and distributes it for free to scientists and researchers, asking them to try it for a firsthand glimpse of schizophrenia.

# "'Gratitude is heaven itself,' said Blake, and I know exactly what he was talking about."

—ALDOUS HUXLEY, following his experiences with mescaline and LSD

But it wasn't scientific accomplishment that sparked broader interest in LSD; it was the revelations of the notoriously reticent screen idol Cary Grant. Grant told a syndicated columnist that he had had a hundred LSD therapy sessions, and that they'd enabled him to turn the concept of "know thyself" into a practical precept. On another occasion, he said, "I don't actually like drugs but LSD did me a lot of good. I think all politicians should take it."

That was an idea that Timothy Leary, then a young adjunct professor of psychology at Harvard, would run with.

## TUNING IN,
## TURNING ON, DROPPING OUT

Leary had had his own psychedelic revelation in the late 1950s when he bought some magic mushrooms on vacation in Mexico. He later described his first trip as a "religious epiphany" that inspired him to set up the Harvard Psilocybin Project upon his return to Cambridge.

In 1962, along with his graduate student Walter Pahnke and fellow faculty member Richard Alpert (who later went to India and returned as the spiritual leader Ram Dass), he launched the landmark Good Friday Experiment at Boston College's Marsh Chapel. Their aim was to compare the power of a pharmacologically induced mystical awakening to a mystical experience induced by religion.

Ten divinity students were given psilocybin, while another ten swallowed niacin, and both groups attended a service led by a charismatic chaplain. The niacin subjects turned red and started sweating. The ten psilocybin recruits wandered around the chapel talking to God. Many had spiritual journeys that mapped to classical mystical experiences.

Twenty-four years later, Rick Doblin, the founder of the Multidisciplinary Association for Psychedelic Studies (MAPS), tracked down nineteen of the original twenty subjects and interviewed them about the salience of their experiences.[10] "The results held up," Doblin told podcaster Joe Rogan.[11] "Eight of the ten still considered their psilocybin mystical experience among the most powerful mystical experiences of their lives. It had motivated them to work in the environmental movement, the women's rights movement, the anti-war movement." To Doblin, this confirmed a long-held suspicion that the hippies had been right: Psychedelics could ignite social change. It took a few more years before he figured out they could play a role in personal transformations, too. But I'm getting ahead of myself.

**1952**—Humphry Osmond and Abram Hoffer begin treating alcoholics with LSD and mescaline. One high dose plus psychotherapy yielded abstinence rates of 50 percent.

**1953**—The CIA launches MK-Ultra, in which thousands of US citizens are given LSD without their knowledge.

**1954**—Aldous Huxley publishes *The Doors of Perception*, in which he describes his experience with mescaline.

When the deans at Harvard learned that Leary and company were using students as experimental subjects, he was reprimanded and eventually fired.* But he was also fired up about the ability of these substances to open people's minds and alter the course of history. "If we could help people plug into the empathy circuits of the brain then positive social change could occur,"[12] he said. Within a few years, he was preaching the gospel of "Turn On, Tune In, Drop Out" to the street. LSD was the quickest route to reach that goal.

Leary was undeniably charismatic, equal parts apostle and adman. Much of his thinking and writing about psychedelics proved prescient, but he made some outrageous claims along the way: LSD could give women hundreds of orgasms; it could "cure" homosexuality as it had with—oops—Allen Ginsberg. But he also believed in the drug's innate ability to reunite people with nature, turn them away from violence and war, and create a more tolerant, creative species that could change the direction of the world one mind at a time. Andrew Weil, who was at Harvard during Leary's tenure, recalls that Leary "envisioned a graduate seminar in which students would take a psychedelic once a week and apply the insights they gained to various social problems. He was absolutely convinced that this was the transformative agent out there . . . He had no sense of the antagonism he would stir up . . . and that's too bad."[13]

# "I turned on five million people and only five thousand ever thanked me."

—TIMOTHY LEARY

The mid-1960s were turbulent years in modern American history, full of disruption, blood, beauty, violence, and shattered assumptions. Vietnam War protests roiled cities; the summer of 1967 saw over 150 race riots. Hippie/drug culture, which rejected middle-class white suburban values, terrified politicians; they viewed the protestors as threats to the pillars of society, or at least to the power structures that held it, and them, in place. For several years, it seemed that every aspect of culture—art, the sciences, fashion, literature, and music—had come under the spell of psychedelics. "There's The Beatles before LSD and then there's The Beatles after LSD," as psychedelic investigator Matthew Johnson so neatly summed it up.[14]

As use of psychedelics spiked, so did problems and fears. Visits to emergency rooms

---

\* In fact, Leary declared himself fired on a TV talk show before Harvard dropped the ax. He was already fashioning himself as a countercultural rebel. "Drugs are the religion of the twenty-first century," he later pronounced.

---

**1955**—R. Gordon Wasson and Allan Richardson are the first Americans to ingest mushrooms in a ceremony led by Maria Sabina in Oaxaca, Mexico.

**1956**—Hungarian chemist Stephen Szára injects DMT and becomes the first person to describe its psychedelic properties.

**1956**—Humphry Osmond coins the word *psychedelic* in a letter to Aldous Huxley.

ticked up,* laying the foundations of an impending public health crisis, or moral crisis, depending on who you were listening to. The media fanned the flames of hysteria with headlines that trumpeted the results of poorly run studies. Some claimed that LSD "broke" chromosomes or drove people to dive off balconies to their deaths. The 1965 Drug Abuse Control Amendments Bill forbade the manufacture and sale of psychedelic drugs; Sandoz, concerned that Delysid could find its way to the black market, stopped production and recalled samples, not only in the US but around the world.

Richard Nixon, who preposterously branded Leary "the most dangerous man in America," went on to win the 1968 presidential election on a "law and order" platform. He launched the first War on Drugs and asked Congress to pass the Controlled Substances Act, which categorized all psychedelics (including cannabis) as Schedule 1 "narcotics." On May 19, 1970, the US doubled down and made psychedelics and all human research into them illegal.

For the ensuing fifty years, science was replaced by a torrent of propaganda about the brain-destroying effects of all psychedelics, with LSD as the main culprit. Albert Hofmann, whom Sandoz executives indirectly blamed** for catalyzing the societal chaos, publicly lamented the "huge wave of an inebriant mania" that turned his wonder child—and all its promise—into his problem child.***

## The Second Wave: Ban

The ostensible strategy behind the so-called War on Drugs was to make drugs harder to get and produce. The DEA put LSD's source material, ergotamine, on its watch list and tracked it with military precision. But even that close level of scrutiny didn't stop underground chemists from pumping out a steady supply, the quality dependent on their skills. Some of these renegade chemists sought to turn a profit, but the most productive of them, according to one insightful 1995 DEA report,[15]**** viewed spreading the benefits of psychedelics as a social calling. All of these chemists did their work clandestinely and on the run. All but one: Dr. Alexander Shulgin.

During the darkest half century of psychedelic repression, Shulgin, who was known as Sasha to his friends, operated as a one-man psychopharmacological research facility in full sight of the law. The documentarian and researcher Hamilton Morris called Shulgin

---

* In 1967, a powerful drug called DOM (aka STP) appeared on the streets of San Francisco. It came in 20 mg tablets, four times more potent than the recommended dosage. Five thousand doses were given away at a "Human Be-In," and hundreds of people experienced extreme trips lasting up to three days. Many ended up in the hospital.

** Toward the end of his working life, Hofmann's requests for salary and title advancements were routinely denied. His retirement gifts included the pitiably modest sum of a hundred thousand Swiss francs and a case of wine, according to Norman Ohler's book *Tripped*.

*** He proclaimed his disappointment in his 1979 autobiography, *LSD: My Problem Child*.

**** While this report is full of fascinating and largely accurate information, it makes a few retrospectively hilarious (but predictable) claims. A notable example is that LSD's "use in psychotherapy largely has been debunked."

---

**1958**—Albert Hofmann isolates the two active agents in mushrooms, psilocybin and psilocin.

**1960**—Alexander Shulgin ingests 400 mg of mescaline sulfate for the first time and changes the direction of his life.

**1962**—Timothy Leary and Richard Alpert conduct the Good Friday (aka Marsh Chapel) Experiment under the auspices of Walter Pahnke.

"the most important psychedelic chemist who has ever lived."[16] The sheer output of his work—three hundred rigorous scientific papers, patents, and books on the chemistry and pharmacology of the compounds he invented—affirms that appraisal.

Shulgin began his career in the 1950s at Dow Chemical Company. After developing a money-minting biodegradable insecticide, he was given the customary $1 bill for the patent but granted free rein to research whatever he liked. In 1960, he took 400 mg of mescaline sulfate, which "unquestionably confirmed the entire direction of my life." He and Dow parted ways in 1966. In the ensuing years, the six-foot-five white-haired wizard, who was beloved for his good cheer and sense of humor,* synthesized 234 psychedelic compounds** in the fully licensed lab he built in a cottage behind his property in Lafayette, California, twenty miles east of San Francisco.

The key word in the previous sentence is *licensed*. In exchange for being an expert witness (usually for the defense) in drug-related trials, Shulgin was granted a DEA research license. He consulted with chemical companies and gave pharmacology lectures to drug agents—he even authored the definitive reference book on controlled substances for law enforcement. But all the while, he was creating new substances, which he tested on himself, his wife, the Jungian psychotherapist Ann Shulgin, and their "research group" of six to eight close friends. In case of a dangerous reaction, Shulgin kept an anticonvulsant on hand, which he used only twice, both times on himself.

Of the hundreds of substances he created over the years, Shulgin's favorite was 2C-B, which he described as "potent, warm, corporeal, and associative." But the one that made the most noise was MDMA.

MDMA had been discovered in 1912 but relegated to history's dustbin. In 1976, a student suggested to Shulgin that he resynthesize it as an alternative to the once popular MDA, which the government had placed into Schedule 1. Shulgin devised a faster synthesis and then tried it on himself. It was instant love. He introduced it to his group, which included a number of West Coast therapists, who in turn began MDMA-assisted psychotherapy with patients. Short acting, music enhancing, and love inducing, MDMA quickly jumped from the couch and to the clubs where it was renamed Ecstasy and fueled the rave scene. Today, Ecstasy, cannabis, and cocaine are the world's most widely used illegal drugs.

Shulgin artfully danced the line between the legitimate and the illicit, but he consistently led with quality science. He described himself as a toolmaker: His instruments allowed people to explore corners of their minds.[17] He was also passionate about the rights of individuals to investigate consciousness without

---

* Shulgin was also a musician who played the viola. A favorite joke from his repertoire: "What's the difference between an orchestra and a bull? The orchestra has horns in the back and its asshole in the front."

** This output rivaled that of many large pharmaceutical companies at the time.

---

**1962**—Howard Lotsof tries ibogaine and after a thirty-three-hour trip learns of its anti-addictive properties.

**1964**—Leary, Alpert, and Ralph Metzner publish *The Psychedelic Experience* and popularize the terms *set* and *setting*.

**1966**—*Life* magazine publishes the cover article "LSD: The Exploding Threat of the Mind Drug That Got Out of Control." Sandoz recalls LSD it had previously distributed.

> # "Our generation is the first, ever, to have made the search for self-awareness a crime if it is done with the use of plants or chemical compounds as the means of opening the psychic doors. But the urge to become aware is always present, and it increases in intensity as one grows older."
>
> —ALEXANDER SHULGIN, *PiHKAL*

interference. The banning of MDMA as a therapeutic agent was a key motivator behind his writing and self-publishing *PiHKAL: A Chemical Love Story* (*PiHKAL* stands for "Phenethylamines I Have Known and Loved") in 1991. The 978-page tome is as eccentric and charming as Shulgin himself. It is divided into two sections. "The Love Story" is a thinly fictionalized account of Sasha's and Ann's love affairs with each other and with drugs. "The Chemical Story" is not a story but rather descriptions of 179 phenethylamines—mescaline, 2C-B, and MDMA the most famous among them—each including "qualitative comments," dosage recommendations, and detailed instructions for synthesis.

It took the DEA a full two years to realize that Shulgin had launched into the public domain a cookbook for the very substances the agency was battling to control. In retaliation, agents raided Shulgin's lab, trampling his precious collection of small peyote cactuses in the fracas. They found no violations (they couldn't arrest him for chemicals found on the premises that had not yet been named or declared illegal!), but they revoked his DEA license and levied a $25,000 fine. (Donations from friends and admirers covered the full amount.)

To the Shulgins, the clampdown was politically motivated. In 1997, they struck back in their ever-gracious way by publishing a second volume, *TiHKAL* (*Tryptamines I Have Known and Loved*), which was similarly structured: Book 1 contained essays by Sasha and Ann; book 2 included recipes for fifty-five tryptamines, including psilocybin, DMT, 5-MeO-DMT, and

---

**1967**—Timothy Leary urges the crowd to "Turn On, Tune In, Drop Out" at a Be-In held in San Francisco's Golden Gate Park.

**1970**—Nixon signs the Controlled Substances Act into law, designating all psychedelics as Schedule 1 substances.

**1971**—Terence McKenna tries psilocybin. Ram Dass publishes *Be Here Now*.

bufotenine. The last section, titled "*Tryptamina Botanica*," included indices to hundreds of plant alkaloids found in nature.

Though it wasn't his intention to become an anti-establishment folk hero, it's difficult to overstate Shulgin's impact on psychedelic culture. Within months of his announcing a new discovery, underground chemists around the world scrambled to pump out gray-market versions. For many, those drugs reaped millions of dollars, but Shulgin never made a penny from sales. He remained committed to keeping his discoveries available for educational purposes. When a friend once recommended he hire offshore chemists to test compounds more quickly, he replied, "Oh, but thinking of new molecules—then creating them—are the greatest delights. One would miss all the fun."

By his death in 2014 at age eighty-eight, Shulgin estimated he had taken four thousand psychedelic journeys. In 2015, the *British Journal of Psychiatry* devoted a special edition to him and Ann; that same year the British Parliament made every substance he listed in *PiHKAL* illegal in one legislative swoop.

## The Third Wave: Boom

If you were a scientist in the 1990s, simply expressing a desire to research psychedelics was the quickest route to career suicide. Professional journals rejected papers on the topic, and universities refused to fund experiments. But two scientists, Rick Strassman and Roland Griffiths—both students of pharmacology and meditation—independently petitioned the authorities to study these forbidden substances. Their efforts were the opening salvo in the professional and public redemption of psychedelics.

Strassman was the first American to legally give a psychedelic to a human being, but not before spending two years fighting his way out of a tangle of red tape.* The object of his inquiry was DMT, a chemical found in plants and the human brain, and which was at one time speculated to be released in flood doses during birth, in dreams, and in near-death experiences.[18]

Roland Griffiths came to prominence by studying caffeine and then lobbying the FDA to list it as an addictive substance. Leveraging his reputation as a scrupulous researcher, he won permission to test psilocybin on cancer patients saddled with crippling end-of-life anxiety. His most cited work was a 2006 study in which high doses of psilocybin were shown to incur mystical experiences in people with depression, which correlated with surprisingly long-term benefits.[19] Both men's work set the stage for other institutions (even the US Department of Defense) to reexamine their anti-psychedelic stances. This "third wave" of psychedelics launched fitfully and with little fanfare, but the results of the research have been breathtaking. And not a minute too soon.

Even before the COVID pandemic, there has been a mental health crisis in North America

---

* The ordeal is dispassionately recounted in his book *DMT: The Spirit Molecule*.

**1976**—Alexander Shulgin develops a new method for synthesizing MDMA.

**1979**—Albert Hofmann publishes *LSD: My Problem Child*; Richard Evans Schultes and Hofmann coauthor and publish *Plants of the Gods*.

**1983**—Ken Nelson, under the pseudonym Albert Most, publishes a tiny print run of *Bufo alvarius: The Psychedelic Toad of the Sonoran Desert*.

that is said to affect some one in five adults.[20] Yet the pharmaceutical industry hasn't come up with any new class of treatments for forty-five years. Nor has there been any new treatment for addiction, not only to opioids, but also to cocaine, nicotine, and alcohol. Anti-opioid medications and programs like Alcohol or Narcotics Anonymous have saved many lives, but they require daily adherence and have a 50 percent fail rate. Psychedelics show similar or better success rates, in many cases after just one or two treatments.

Psychedelics are now being studied to battle other confounding diseases such as OCD, anxiety, PTSD, cluster headaches, and anorexia nervosa, the deadliest mental illness of all.[21] LSD for pain? You haven't heard about that? Funny, the scientific community has known of LSD's analgesic properties since the 1970s. Likewise, you may not have known that ibogaine, psilocybin, and MDMA are all being used conjointly with therapy to treat athletes, law enforcement, and soldiers suffering from traumatic brain injuries or PTSD. Marcus Capone, an ex–Navy SEAL who struggled with incapacitating PTSD for years, told me that the combined ibogaine/5-MeO-DMT treatments he received in Mexico "changed my life and saved my life." He and his wife, Amber, have since started VETS (Veterans Exploring Treatment Solutions), a nonprofit that raises money to send other veterans to offshore ibogaine clinics for treatment.

Once research on adults shows safety, the FDA could possibly consider testing psychedelics with adolescents, who are also struggling with addiction and depression at alarming rates. The psychedelic investigator Matthew Johnson, best known for his studies on tobacco addiction, says that while there's risk in exposing developing brains to psychedelics, both illnesses are spiking in younger populations, so the bigger risk may be in not testing those potential treatments.[22]

Of course, the big questions are: How do all of these different compounds effectively treat such a vast and seemingly distinct variety of differing conditions? What commonalities underlie these diseases that we don't yet understand? How can one drug that was developed in a lab as an anesthetic (ketamine) and one that comes from plants in the Amazon (ayahuasca) and one from equatorial Africa (iboga) all work to alleviate both depression and addiction? Early evidence suggests that psychedelics rearrange people's brains in ways that allow them to escape negative thought loops and eventually thrive. Over three hundred clinical trials are now up and running in search of some answers.

Governments are following suit, if upticks in funding are any indication. In July 2023, Health Canada granted $3 million to study psilocybin psychotherapy for depression.[23] In 2021, the US National Institutes of Health kicked in $4 million to study psilocybin-assisted therapy for tobacco addiction. Australia legalized psilocybin- and MDMA-assisted psychotherapies in late 2023, and practitioners from around the world were heading there hoping to lead the change. In 2020, DARPA (the Defense Advanced Research Projects Agency,

**1985**—MDMA is put in Schedule 1.

**1986**—MAPS is founded by Rick Doblin.

**1990-95**—Rick Strassman studies DMT at the University of New Mexico.

**1993**—David Nichols launches the Heffter Research Institute to promote research with the classic psychedelics.

part of the US Department of Defense) allotted $27 million to engineer a psychedelic that treats PTSD without the pacifist "side effects" that the trip famously induces.[24] The DoD wants soldiers to heal their trauma without putting down their arms.

There are more than two thousand ketamine clinics in the US today; MAPS estimates that there will be over five thousand psychedelic centers for depression by 2027, if the government doesn't slide into another backlash.

Recreationally, use continues to climb. The value of the US magic mushroom market is projected to hit $95 billion in 2028,[25] on a par with baby food and more than a hundred times that of M&M'S. Every weekend an estimated 750,000 people in Britain use MDMA. That's an order of magnitude larger than the estimated ten to twenty thousand psilocybin users. Oregon and Colorado have legalized supervised psychedelic use,[26] and a few dozen cities and municipalities are following suit. All are experiments worth watching. The Caribbean nation of St. Vincent and the Grenadines is legalizing the cultivation of psilocybin and other visionary plants, angling to become a global supplier ahead of the impending demand.

Venture capital is bankrolling start-ups that are deploying artificial intelligence to compress ten years of drug development into eighteen months. A good number of these baby biopharma start-ups are tinkering with existing molecular structures to create "pseudodelics" that deliver powerful changes in brain chemistry without the trip. Other start-ups are eyeing novel substances that could give healthy people a cognitive edge in learning, memory, and decision making. Ethical issues aside—and plenty of dystopian scenarios come to mind when imagining who will control these mind-bending chemicals—the psychedelic boom, and all of the messy complications that accompany any boom, is underway.

There's a long way to go before this third wave crests. As psychiatrist and psychedelic researcher Dr. Ben Sessa says, "Psychedelics today are where twentieth-century medicine was before the discovery of antibiotics. We're classifying illnesses and identifying symptoms but still lacking insight into how these substances work."[27] The next chapter explores what these medicines do in the brain to enable such magnificent changes.

## CODA

Toward the end of their lives, Alexander Shulgin and his wife, Ann, lived modestly, drawing income from a small stock portfolio, Social Security checks, and the rent that two phone companies paid to build cell towers on their land. Family members and friends have launched a nonprofit to preserve the property and open it as a retreat center. Learn more about this trailblazing couple and see the farm at shulginfoundation.org.

On the day of his death, November 22, 1963, Aldous Huxley, riven with laryngeal cancer, scribbled a note to his wife, Laura, who was by his bedside. It said: "LSD 100 micrograms, intramuscular." He died tripping, as the assas-

---

**1995**—Erowid online drug directory is founded by Earth and Fire Erowid. It grows to sixty thousand pages.

**1998**—Amanda Feilding launches the Beckley Foundation in the UK to pioneer psychedelic research and advocate for evidence-informed drug policy reform.

**1998**—Swiss researcher Franz Vollenweider shows that psilocybin produces its psychedelic effect by activating the 5-HT2A serotonin receptor.

sination of John F. Kennedy was broadcast on television.

Albert Hofmann took his final dose of LSD at age ninety-nine. At a 2006 symposium in Basel, Switzerland, celebrating his one hundredth birthday, he told the audience, "I believe that LSD told me, 'Introduce me to the world, so that I will not be forgotten.'"[28] The thunderous applause indicated that the crowd was in full agreement. Hofmann died at age 102 on April 29, 2008, sixty-five years and ten days after the date of his first acid trip.

## WHAT IS A MYSTICAL EXPERIENCE?

In the early 1960s, physician Walter Pahnke surveyed the literature of mysticism in the world's major religions and extracted six common themes. He removed the symbols specific to each religion and created the Mystical Experience Questionnaire that is still used in clinical research today.

The six components are:
1. A searing sense of the sacred: that you have met Cosmic Consciousness, the Infinite, the Source of All Being, God, whatever you wish to call it.
2. A noetic quality: The experience is imbued with meaning or a sense of some ultimate reality. You have somehow encountered the foundation of existence.
3. A deeply felt positive mood: joy, ecstasy, blessedness, peace, tenderness, gentleness, tranquility, awe . . .
4. Ineffability: What you experience is beyond words or limitless.
5. A paradox: You accept the coexistence of seemingly mutually exclusive states or concepts: Both/And vs. Either/Or.
6. A unitary consciousness that transcends time and space and blurs the boundaries between self and other, subject and object.

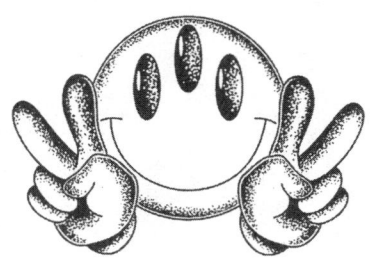

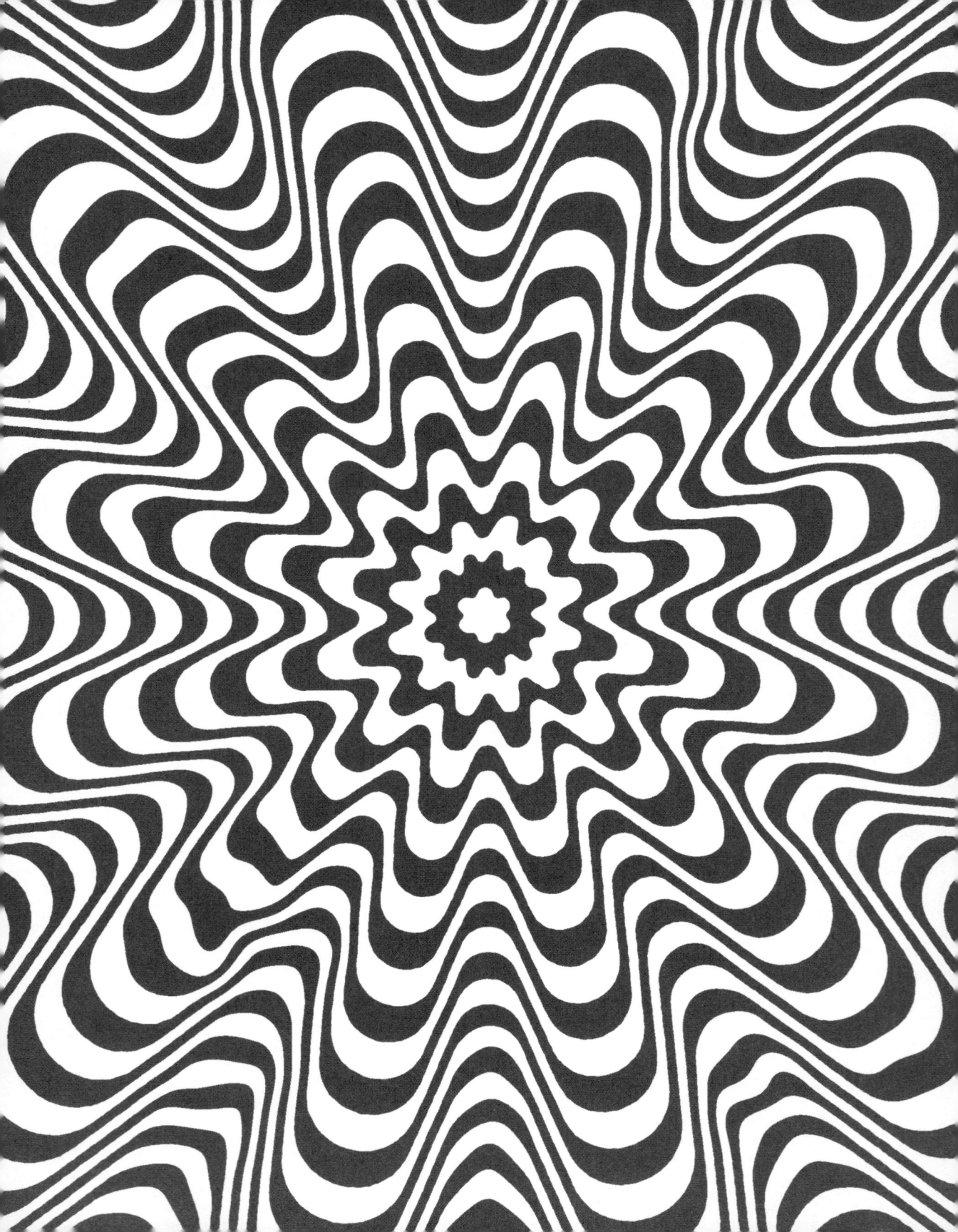

# CHAPTER 3

# UNDER THE HOOD

## THE BRAIN SCIENCE OF PSYCHEDELICS

--------------------------------------------------------------

*We can say these chemicals bind to serotonin 2A receptors and they activate glutamate circuits ... but we really just don't have a clue about how all of that connects to what is happening in the psyche.[1]*

DAVID E. PRESTI, professor of neurobiology at UC Berkeley and the author
of *Foundational Concepts in Neuroscience: A Brain-Mind Odyssey*

What are psychedelics doing in our brains? And what can we do to ensure we have better trips?

Anyone who has ever taken a psychedelic has likely grappled with these questions. Until recently, philosophers and psychoanalysts tried to provide answers, but they lacked the tools for deep investigation. Today it's neuroscientists (or psychologists with fMRI or MEG[*] scanning machines) who are leading the inquiries, so that's who I turned to first.

Brain scans are the tools most commonly used to investigate the brain's landscape and activity. Subjects are given a shot of psilocybin[**] and slid into fMRI machines with electrodes attached to their skulls. Scientists measure the increases or decreases in blood flow to infer the neural activity and mental states caused by the psychedelic. It's common to hear scientists say things like, "MDMA decreases activity in the amygdala, the brain area responsible for the fear response. This

---

* fMRI, functional magnetic resonance imaging, measures the small changes in blood flow that occur with brain activity. MEG, magnetoencephalography, is another imaging technology that identifies brain activity by measuring small magnetic fields produced in the brain.

** A trip from injected psilocybin lasts for only forty-five minutes, not the five or six hours it lasts when orally consumed as a mushroom.

---

| **1999**—Roland Griffiths initiates research at Johns Hopkins studying psilocybin for end-of-life anxiety. | **2006**—Griffiths's landmark paper, "Psilocybin Can Occasion Mystical-Type Experiences Having Substantial and Sustained Personal Meaning and Spiritual Significance," is published in *Psychopharmacology*. | **2011**—5-MeO-DMT is made a Schedule 1 drug. |

allows people to process their experiences with less fear.["]*

fMRI is also used to track activity in neural networks, which are a group of interconnected brain regions that are theorized to produce different types of cognition. If you've read *How to Change Your Mind* by Michael Pollan, you may recall that psychedelics reduce activity in the default mode network (DMN), which is thought to control ruminative thinking and contribute to our conception of "self." Originally, scientists supposed that psychedelics would amp up activity in this part of the brain, but fMRI showed the opposite—that psychedelics cause this network to quiet down. This led to the theory that the DMN becomes overly active in people who are depressed or suffering from mental illnesses. More negative thinking leads to more rumination, which leads to a biological entrenchment of neural patterns in the brain. Think of those negative thought patterns as akin to cross-country ski tracks that become more rutted in snow over time. Psychedelics are thought to "loosen the snow" and discharge those habitual dark thoughts, giving people a new perspective on their problems and the world.

Other studies by Franz Vollenweider's lab in Switzerland, using a different technology, support the idea that the visual and other perceptual changes are caused by dysregulation in the thalamus (or, more correctly, thalamic circuits).[2]

The thalamus is a brain region that filters the barrage of sensory information coming at us in all waking moments; it "decides" what to transfer to conscious awareness. A more exact version of Huxley's reducing valve, the thalamus literally takes all the information from our senses and reduces it down to a manageable fraction of the total. This is hugely important because, without this "gating," as it's called, the overload would incapacitate us, making us unable to focus our attention or function.

Psychedelics send the thalamus, the gatekeeper of our senses, on vacation. Whether or not this constitutes a distortion of reality or presents a truer picture of what surrounds us is unknowable; no matter, the thalamus dysregulation model makes a lot of intuitive sense. It helps to bridge the gap between explanation and experience.

Brain scans give us a peek inside our brains, the most dauntingly complex thing in the universe. But there's not much that we explorers (or therapists, for that matter) can do with a thalamus or a default mode network. While brain scans may be revealing, it's unlikely that they're giving us the full picture of what's going on under the hood. At least that's what studies with octopuses on MDMA suggest.

---

* You'll read statements like that in this book as well. Tying mental states to brain structures as a result of scanning has become de rigueur in psychedelic science today. But while it's true that the amygdala is involved in fear, it is also involved in many other mental activities. This is why some neuroscientists object to equating snapshots of neural function with mental states. They consider it a gross oversimplification.

---

**2014**—Robin Carhart-Harris uses fMRI to produce a map of the brain's internal communications under psychedelics.

**2016**—NYU studies show that one dose of psilocybin combined with therapy relieves anxiety and depression for over six months.

**2018**—David Olson shows that LSD and DMT increase neural growth in petri dishes, suggesting that they "repair" brains in people with mood and anxiety disorders.

## Octopuses on Ecstasy

Gül (pronounced *Gool*) Dölen is a Turkish American neuroscientist who in 2023 became the Bob and Renee Parsons* Endowed Chair in psychedelics, psychology, and neuroscience at the University of California–Berkeley. She is considered one of the leading researchers in the field of psychedelics. (Though she is now at Berkeley, much of her research was conducted at Johns Hopkins.)

In college, Dölen developed her own major, Comparative Perspectives on the Mind, a blend of Eastern philosophy, neuroscience, linguistics, and art. She went on to earn her MD and her PhD from Brown University and MIT, but she never practiced medicine. It was neuroscience that compelled her, especially investigating what philosophers call the "hard question of consciousness." Based on her past work investigating the pathophysiology of diseases such as autism and schizophrenia, she had a suspicion that something else was happening on a more molecular level in the brain that her colleagues' scans weren't picking up. It is one of the main reasons she gave octopuses molly.

Most MDMA studies are performed on mammals whose brains structurally resemble those of humans. But octopus brains are nothing like human brains—they're more akin to slugs. Our last common ancestor was 650 million years ago—that predates the dinosaurs—so when Dölen bathed her octopuses in water laced with Ecstasy, "there was a good chance nothing was going to happen."

If anything, Dölen presumed that once dosed, the octopuses would speed around the tank in a frenzy or stand at attention, since MDMA is structurally similar to methamphetamine. And at high doses, that's exactly what occurred. But as doses were lowered to correspond to what humans take, the octopuses relaxed, doing backflips and engaging in a floaty eight-arm water ballet. They became docile and remarkably social. In contrast with what *My Octopus Teacher* might lead you to believe, octopuses are aggressively antisocial creatures. Except for brief mating periods, they're more prone to attacking fellow octopods than cuddling with them. That's why everyone in Dölen's lab was surprised when the octopuses on Ecstasy broke through a barrier to nuzzle up to one another. This "socializing" was a 180-degree change in behavior.[3]

What the findings indicate is that the original conclusions based on scans of human brains on psychedelics may have led researchers in the wrong direction. MDMA may appear to be dampening activity in the amygdala or activating the thalamus in mammalian brains, but the octopus brain differs from the human brain in that these regions do not exist. For MDMA to have the same effect on humans as it does on octopuses, it must be acting on a common biological structure or function shared by the two.

---

* Bob Parsons founded GoDaddy, among other enterprises. He has a son with autism. Dölen's earlier work focused on critical periods and a form of autism called Fragile X syndrome.

# "Psychedelics restore the ability to be amazed by all of the mystery and magic that a child experiences all the time."

—GÜL DÖLEN

And what octopus brains share with human brains is a nearly identical serotonin transporter, a protein that recycles serotonin (a neurotransmitter that's key to regulating mood) by moving it back into the cell from the synapse.

Dölen's findings suggest that psychedelics aren't simply altering the connections within and between certain brain areas. Instead, they are working on a deeper, molecular level to open so-called critical periods of learning.

## OLD MICE, NEW TRICKS

In 1935, Konrad Lorenz observed that baby snow geese learn to recognize and respond to their mother forty-eight hours after hatching in a process known as imprinting. They follow Mom around,* studying her every move, learning how to feed, how to vocalize with their fellow goslings, and other basic survival skills. Lorenz called this the critical period in which the brain is chemically sensitized to absorbing massive amounts of information in a finite period of time.** He won the Nobel Prize for the discovery.

It turns out that, just like young goslings, young humans also have critical periods for learning the skills they need to survive, and once a particular critical period closes, learning that skill becomes more difficult. We see evidence of this in that it's easier to learn a language or ride a bike earlier in life. Babies who are deprived of touch have a hard time establishing intimate relations as adults because their critical period closed before those emotional ties were established.

Dölen and other neuroscientists suspect there are as many critical periods as there are brain functions, and they theorize that there is a critical period for every skill we develop. But all critical periods close for good reason. "Living in a world where you're highly sensitized and paying attention to everything around you is emotionally and energetically costly," says Dölen. "At some point, you want a stable representation of the world that is not changing as much; that's why critical periods close." It's also one reason

---

\* When deprived of their mother, the baby goslings began to follow Lorenz, which was what initially aroused his curiosity about their behavior.

\*\* Some people use the word *neuroplasticity* interchangeably with *critical period*. Dölen is very clear that they are not the same. All learning causes neuroplasticity, she says. Critical periods are finite.

---

**2023**—Australia legalizes MDMA-assisted therapy for PTSD and psilocybin-assisted therapy for depression.

**August 9, 2024**—The FDA stuns researchers by declining to approve the use of MDMA-assisted therapy for PTSD in the US. After decades of clinical studies and tens of millions spent, the FDA requested further studies on safety and efficacy.

adults develop habits that allow us to perform many tasks efficiently or on autopilot. It would be highly inefficient to constantly be learning and relearning the same thing repeatedly. The downside is that habits can make the magic of the world seem a little less magical as we age.

In a follow-up experiment to the octopus study, Dölen dosed adult mice with MDMA. She wanted to see if she could open a critical period for social behavior and how long it would stay open once the cuddly effects of MDMA wore off.[4] Older mice are far less social than juveniles. Just like people, they enjoy being surrounded by a hundred other "friends" when they're young, but they value their alone time as adults. Surprisingly, for two weeks following MDMA, the adult mice continued to snuggle with other mice just like teenagers.[*] In further tests with LSD, ibogaine, ketamine, and psilocybin—psychedelics that are all far less social than MDMA—the old mice continued cuddle puddling, sometimes for weeks after the drug effects ended.

"We're in year four of trying to figure out this mechanism, but this study suggests that *all* psychedelics reopen a critical period and they do it whether they are prosocial drugs like MDMA, or hallucinogenics like psilocybin or LSD, or dissociatives like ketamine, or dream-inducing oneirogens like ibogaine. All psychedelics do it. *And that tells us that the prosocial character of MDMA is a red herring; instead, all psychedelics are putting the brain in an altered state[**] which we think is the same as an open critical period.[***]* It's what all psychedelics share in common. The ability to open critical periods coheres the category."

Dölen isn't yet sure how this works, but she has an inkling. By using an advanced whole cell patch technology, her lab has been able to measure the activity inside the neurons of cells extracted from mouse brains. These intraneural investigations showed that psychedelics are actually resetting the molecular structure inside cells. "When psychedelics hit the brain, they sit in a variety of receptors for an unusually long time. This may be sending a signal to the brain that something is abnormal here, something is frozen, and that sets off a biochemical reaction that tells it to reestablish new connections." A psychedelic trip is like a biochemical "resetting of the router in our brains," is how she describes it. And it parallels the opening of a critical period.

"It doesn't have to do with my default mode network or my amygdala," she adds, contradicting the countervailing wisdom. "By reopening critical periods, psychedelics enable the brain to get back to that state where it's receptive to the world, like a child, and open to learning new things."

Interestingly, it appears the critical period remains open far longer than the effects of the trip last. Further studies on mice have correlated the length of each psychedelic journey with the length of time each critical period remains open. It's not the strength of the dose driving this correlation. It's the length of the journey. A ketamine trip lasts thirty to forty-five minutes; the critical period closes two to four days later. MDMA and psilocybin journeys

---

[*] This type of bonding does not occur with non-psychedelic drugs. After the high of cocaine wears off, mice get cranky and isolate just as we humans do.

[**] Had Dölen put mice through a visual experiment rather than a social learning one, she suspects their visual critical period would have opened.

[***] Emphasis added.

last about six hours; the critical period closes at two weeks. LSD is eight hours. The critical period is three weeks. Ibogaine lasts thirty-six to seventy-two hours, and the upper limit of that critical period is yet to be determined.

| DRUG[5] | LENGTH OF TRIP | LENGTH OF OPEN CRITICAL PERIOD |
|---|---|---|
| Ketamine | 30–60 minutes | 2–4 days |
| Psilocybin | 3–6 hours | 2 weeks |
| MDMA | 3–6 hours | 2 weeks |
| LSD | 6–10 hours | 3 weeks |
| Ibogaine | 72 hours | > 4 weeks |

## THE CONTEXT DRIVES THE OUTCOME

In Dölen's model, the psychedelic is the catalyst that opens the brain to new learning, but what you learn depends on the context in which the drug is administered. Taking MDMA at a rave won't have any effect on your PTSD, "but in the company of a supportive therapist over time, the same drug permits people to undertake the cognitive reappraisal needed to heal," she says. This is why the psychedelic aspects of a trip, and what bookends it, may be more important than most people currently think. The intention you set prior to a trip primes the neurons in the brain that hold memories or feelings to become malleable again. The psychedelic biochemically opens the critical period, which allows people to wander down the rabbit holes of their minds, stumbling across old memories or trauma and appraising them anew. In follow-up sessions,

## THE DOWNSIDE OF OPENING A CRITICAL PERIOD WITH PSYCHEDELICS

If the inputs are not tightly controlled and monitored, people on psychedelics can be damaged or destabilized. The example most often cited is that of Charles Manson, who bombarded his cult followers with high doses of LSD and filled their very open minds with murderous ideas. Anthropological studies are full of examples of psychedelic plants being used to encourage fighting, violence, and war. Hacking critical periods with psychedelics can be a dangerous pursuit if the inputs aren't controlled. The context can be more powerful than the drug.

people talk about their insights, if there were any, and therapeutic support helps them figure out how to integrate the insights into their lives.[*]

The model is not dissimilar to what happens to Neo in *The Matrix*, the 1999 film that psychonauts have been obsessively dissecting for decades. Neo takes the red pill, which brings him into the Matrix. Once there, a video is downloaded into his system, but he doesn't instantly become a jujitsu master. He first must train and practice before he can take down his enemies. The red pill = the psychedelic. The download = the trip. The training = support and integration.

---

* There are numerous complicated neurological processes underpinning memory retrieval, involving the extracellular matrix and other structures, which can't be explained in this book.

## THE DEPRIVATION CONNECTION: MYSTICAL EXPERIENCES AND HALLUCINATIONS EXPLAINED

When neuroscientists are preparing animals to study critical periods, they put them in deprivation boxes to cut them off from the senses they are trying to test. Mice are put in a dark box for days before they are exposed to light; the exposure opens a visual critical period. To open an auditory critical period, animals' ears are plugged before exposing them to sound.

It was during the isolation of the pandemic that Dölen herself made the connection between deprivation and the mystical revelations that people commonly experience under the influence of a psychedelic. "The mystics lived alone in isolation in a cave, or they walked on their knees across the desert for forty days, or they fasted for long periods of time. All are states of deprivation and we think that this kind of deprivation also opens critical periods just as a psychedelic does," she says. "Zen Buddhists sit in silence trying to undo layers of ego to achieve what they call 'beginner's mind.' If you were looking for a neurobiological definition of beginner's mind, it would be a critical period."

The power of deprivation to induce hallucinations and mystical experiences has been known for millennia. Contemporary neurological studies[6] show that visual deprivation in healthy humans (five days with a blindfold) caused hallucinations in 77 percent of participants.

"If you conceptualize depression as a lasting habit of thinking about the world or yourself in a negative way, then the real utility of the psychedelic is to break that habit and allow you to create new thinking that enables you to see the world with a new, updated sense of what's possible," is how Dölen explains it. PTSD is similar. "The traumatizing event [such as surviving rape] causes people to close down. That's an adaptive response that may have saved someone's life in that moment, but over time it interferes with their ability to trust, form bonds, and engage in the world. If the psychedelic can open a critical period so you can revisit those maladaptive responses without the threat, you may be able to learn to stand up to your rapist and confront your fear from the stronger version of yourself today."

### MASTER KEYS

Scientists have long been interested in reopening critical periods in adults, but they have feared that doing so might disrupt the neural and chemical connections that hold our memories, habits, and histories—the accumulated knowledge that distinguishes you from me—in place. But Dölen suspects that under controlled conditions, psychedelics might be used to encourage such reopenings, not only for mental disturbances but for physical disabilities, too. Her next experiments will test her theories by seeing if psychedelics can be used to restore physical function in people who have lost limb movement following a stroke.*

Typically, stroke victims regain some function in the first three months of recovery; after that, improvement flatlines because that critical period has closed. Dölen's lab will pair psychedelics with a new type of 3D physical therapy to investigate if they can return people to that early post-stroke period of improvement even if their stroke occurred years prior.

It's commonly said that psychedelic therapy "rewires" the brain, but until Dölen's research, no one could offer a satisfying explanation for how this entire class of compounds that have such a short duration of effects can produce transformations that extend for months or, in some cases, years.

Ancient sages, curanderos, and ayahuasqueros have a saying: "Once the trip has ended, the real work begins." Neuroscience may finally be catching up to them.

## Taking the Trip Out of Psychedelics (or the "Fun" Out of Fungi)

If you've read anything about psychedelics in the last decade, you've probably heard that they work by sparking neuroplasticity. The term *plasticity* refers to the brain's ability to change in response to environmental inputs. Different from a critical period (in which a vast amount of learning occurs for a brief, limited period of time), plasticity is the way the brain responds to everyday stimulation and learns in a more routine way. Psychedelics have been shown to accelerate plasticity within hours.

There's nothing new about the concept of human and animal brains changing in response to everyday experience. Everything we learn sparks neuroplasticity. But in the last few years, the word *plasticity* has entered the realm of psychedelic psychobabble. Its definition changes depending on who's using it. Psychologists use it metaphorically to describe more flexible ways of thinking. Chemists use it to refer to morphological changes in cells. The chemist David Olson, who runs his own lab at the University of California–Davis, is using the word to describe a new class of psychedelics he's trying to engineer that creates neuronal growth without the trip. He calls them psychoplastogens.

In Olson's model, some mental illnesses are caused by atrophied neurons in the prefrontal cortex of the brain. If psychoplastogens can get those old neurons up and running or spark some new neuronal connections, they might be able to alleviate depression, PTSD, even bipolar disorder.

To envision this, picture two neighboring trees. The branches that grow upward are comparable to the dendrites of a neuron, and the leaves are the synapses between them. A healthy brain has a full canopy of leaves that touch each other and facilitate communication among trees. But many brain disorders resemble trees in winter: Fallen leaves and barren branches break up the canopy and make communication impossible.[7] Olson is betting that psychoplastogens can regrow those neuronal arbors and reestablish lost synaptic connectivity—and

---

* Giving psychedelics to people who've had strokes will involve its own set of complications!

the venture capital world is supporting him. Delix Therapeutics, the biotech company he has cofounded, has raised $10 million in investment capital to reengineer psychedelics that can spark neuronal growth without the inconvenient side effects of the trip.

Skeptics, and there are many, say that growing neurons in petri dishes can't be compared to how neurons grow when they are bathed in the complex soup of proteins, sugars, and other chemicals in the brain. It's like trying to sprout seeds without water or soil. Other critics argue that not all brain plasticity is beneficial. Cocaine creates massive growth of new dendrites—the "branches" that sprout when healthy neurons are growing—but they also lead to deeper cravings for more coke all the time. People with autism spectrum disorder have a form of hyperplasticity that causes behavioral and emotional challenges (but may also be responsible for some of the superskills they display). What's more, there's little evidence that neuroplasticity without the learning that comes from the trip or the follow-up therapy has any beneficial effect on mental illnesses. Rick Doblin of MAPS, who has devoted almost forty years to shepherding MDMA-assisted psychotherapy through the FDA, calls the pursuit of a trip-free chemical intervention a pipe dream. "The content of the trip provides a lot of meaning for people and people are meaning makers," he says.

My more cynical side tells me that a trip-free pill that can be patented and that comes without the hours-long trip or additional hours of therapy is a solution that some patients might like, and that Big Pharma would love. My less cynical side knows there is a precedent for such moon shots. In 2006, people suffering from cluster headaches (also known as suicide headaches because the pain is so excruciating) began noticing that LSD brought them relief. Scientists in Switzerland were brought in to do testing, but since LSD is illegal, subjects were given 2-bromo-LSD, an LSD analog that caused a biological action without the trip.[8] The non-psychedelic LSD was more effective, and it is popular among cluster headache sufferers today.

As of this writing, venture capital is funding several dozen start-ups that are racing to tweak or patent non-psychedelic analogs. It's a safe bet that VC firms are more interested in financial outcomes than patient outcomes, but maybe the two won't be mutually exclusive. Any new drug that treats intractable diseases and relieves suffering is worth a shot, moon shots included.

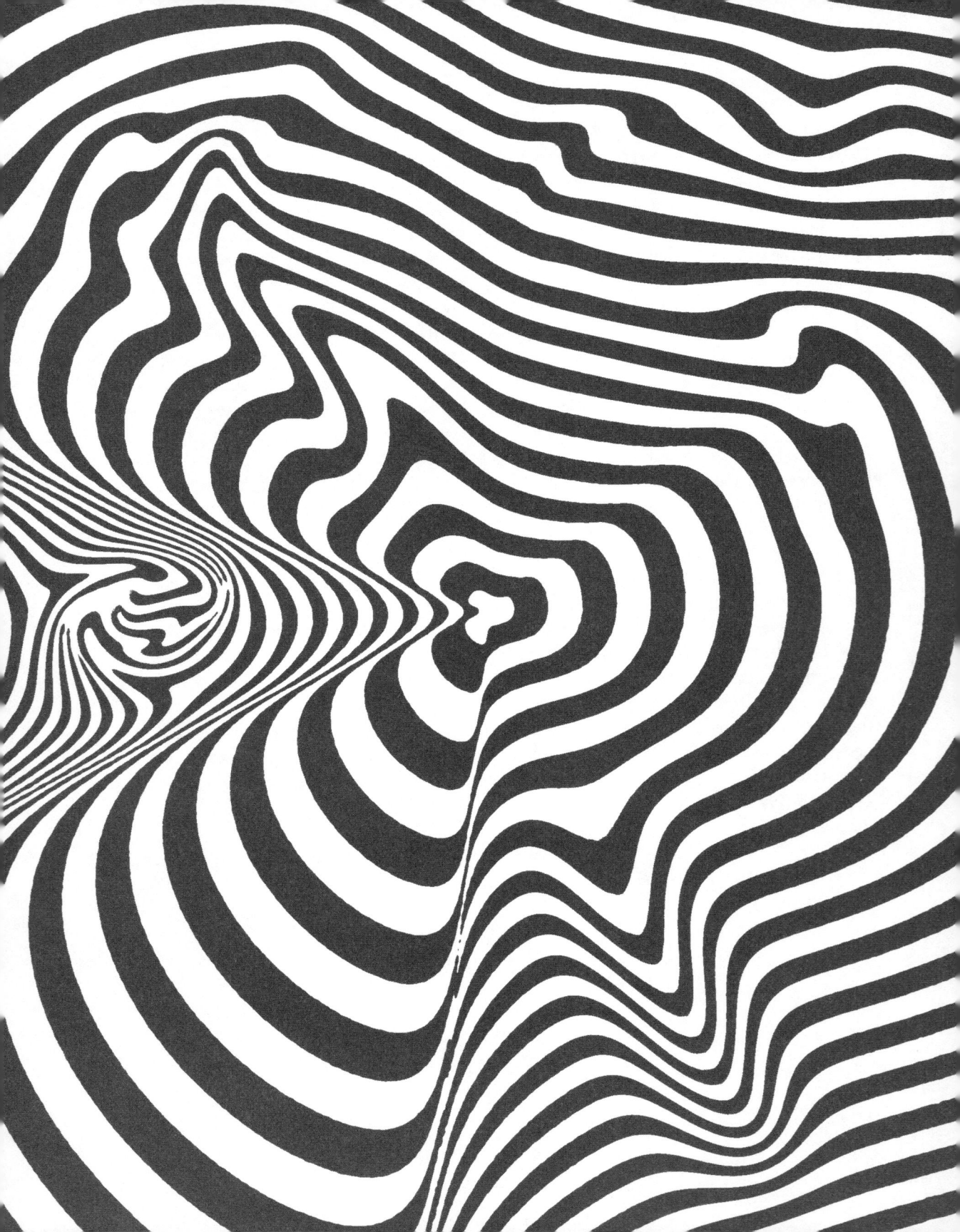

# CHAPTER 4

# HAVE A GREAT TRIP

## FLIGHT PATH, TAKEOFF, LANDING

------------------------------------------------------

Psychedelic drugs are simply instruments, like microscopes, telescopes, and telephones. The biologist does not sit with eye permanently glued to the microscope; he goes away and works on what he has seen.

ALAN WATTS, *The Joyous Cosmology*

In 1967, Timothy Leary and the psychologist Ralph Metzner published the landmark essay "Programming the Psychedelic Experience." They compared shamanic rituals across cultures with their own extensive knowledge and determined that psychedelics "put people in a state of delicate suggestibility" that sparked a period of "increased reactivity to stimulation from without and within." Their conclusion: By patterning the inputs, voyagers "could steer awareness toward useful spaces of the mind and navigate that evanescent flux of sensation and perception toward a place of ecstatic illumination."

While some believe that psychedelics work independently of where you are, who you're with, or how you approach the trip, it has long been accepted that these "inputs" (intention and context) can be orchestrated to achieve more meaningful outcomes. Controlling every aspect of a journey may be impossible, but there

are ways to launch it in the right direction and smooth some of the bumps along the way.

In 1966, Willis Harman, an electrical engineer, and psychologist James Fadiman, both at Stanford University, launched an experiment to test the effects of psychedelics on creative problem-solving. They invited twenty-six scientists, artists, and engineers to a guided mescaline* experiment at the International Foundation for Advanced Study, their "privately funded research facility" housed in offices above a beauty parlor in Menlo Park, California. They had a USDA permit to perform psychedelic studies (not uncommon at the time). The subjects were selected exclusively from the nascent field of computer technology and engineering. There were no women, as women weren't welcome in those industries at the time.

Harman and Fadiman asked volunteers to bring to the session a thorny work problem

---

\* The researchers used mescaline instead of LSD because the FDA insisted on examining their Sandoz LSD, which could have delayed the experiment indefinitely.

that they had been unable to solve but in which they were emotionally invested. Each subject was dosed with 200 mg mescaline (the equivalent of 100 mcg of LSD) and then left alone to trip. After a few hours and some lunch, they set to work on their problems. Some stayed long into the night. The results were striking to the subjects and the researchers alike. Many had flashes of intellectual intuition; they were able to restructure the problem in a larger context; they had heightened empathy with external processes and with people; and they were more able to visualize solutions. Their performance on psychometric tests improved, and a high percentage solved equations and problems that had previously eluded them. Curiously, none had even an inkling of a so-called mystical experience.

From this experiment, Fadiman theorized that psychedelics could provide a steely clarity of focus but do not inspire a global transformation; instead, they operate in the object of your attention. Unfortunately, the study took place on the same day the Feds banned psychedelic research. Actually, it occurred the day after the ban, but prior to enforcement, so it was never replicated. However, in the years since the Stanford experiment, neuroscience has verified that bringing thoughts into conscious awareness activates engrams* that encode memories. Today, there's a consensus that:

- A psychedelic used in a therapeutic setting will grant increased awareness of nonconscious personal or emotional issues.
- A spiritual intention will increase chances of having a transcendent

experience that could cause you to reevaluate your place in the universe.
- Focusing on an intellectual problem that you care about solving before you trip may yield cognitive insights.

This research, and many other studies, reinforces the notion that "intention" and "setting" are essential to (but not determinants of) a successful and fruitful journey.

## Intention: Logging Your Flight Path

Articulating an intention before you trip can be considered an opening statement in the dialogue between you and the psychedelic, putting you and the medicine on the same flight path so you move in the same direction during the voyage.

Your intention can be an aim or goal you hold for the duration of the experience and the continuation of your insight or healing. It can focus your mind ahead of your trip and serve as an anchor to return to if things get scary.

Sometimes images or thoughts that occur during a trip connect directly to your intention. Other times the connection is fuzzier. Still, recalling your intention can help you understand why the experience unfolded as it did or what it was trying to tell you.

Coming back to your intention during your trip can recenter you if you feel challenged, unsure, or resistant to what's coming up. It can be a reassuring home base to which you can return.

Daan Keiman, a psychedelic chaplain in the Buddhist tradition who has been leading journeys for fifteen years, suggests using the familiar mantra "Trust, let go, be open." You can come

---

* An engram is a collection of neurons across brain regions that store memories. Most memories are inactive until specific events activate them.

back to it during a difficult period and it doubles as a handy teaching device for working with psychedelics.

## TIPS FOR SETTING
## YOUR INTENTION

1. Make your intention open-ended, not prescriptive. "Teach me about my joy" as opposed to "I want to find joy."

2. Stay humble and affirmative. Rather than "I want . . . " or "I need . . . ," try "I'm in the process of . . . ," "I am working on . . . "

3. Avoid focusing your intention on something dark or scary; that's an invitation to a bad trip. Instead of "I want to revisit a childhood trauma," make it "Help me rediscover my younger self."

4. Let simplicity be your guide. Dimitri Mugianis, an experienced psychedelic practitioner and harm reduction specialist recommends setting a clear intention, but one that allows some room for exploration. Something like, "I want to be a more loving person to myself and others."

5. Avoid making the focus of your intention too narrow. Mugianis says, "Any intention that is too constricting can result in more self-judgment." For example, if your intention is "I'm going to lose twenty pounds," try focusing instead on the broader feeling you're hoping to achieve or what's getting in the way of that, such as "I'd like to better understand my relationship to food."

6. Keep your intention focused on your present circumstances. Ido Cohen, a clinical psychologist and the founder of The Integration Circle in the Bay Area, counsels that focusing closely on where you are is usually a better place to begin than aiming for somewhere you hope to be. A client of his came in wanting "to see God." A bit of probing revealed more pressing concerns about what was happening in her life: She was feeling lonely, working fifteen hours a day, and her health was in ruins. He suggested she try to merge her present with the wish. She decided to bring her suffering to God and ask for help.

7. Once you set an intention, let it go and allow the psychedelic to open a door. Put your effort into the things you can control.

## WHAT AN INTENTION
## SHOULD NOT BE

An intention isn't a requirement or a demand such as "Either I have this experience/sensation/insight or the session didn't work." You can't insist your way to healing or illumination. Nor does an intention have to involve deep emotional work or an internal quest for healing. Sometimes all that is needed for a satisfying session is "Let me stay open to what is revealed."

## WHAT IF YOUR INTENTION
## DOESN'T HAPPEN?

Despite your best efforts at mapping a flight path, the psychedelic may have other ideas for where your trip will go. This can be disappointing or baffling, but there is value in looking for alternative ways of interpreting your experience. If your intention was "Show me what I need to heal," and

**"You may not get the trip you want, but you get the trip you need."**
This is a well-worn and often annoying cliché in psychedelic circles (especially when someone says it to you after you've just come through hell), but some clichés are born in truth.

Karla was on the brink of a big career change but uncertain which direction she should head. She joined an ayahuasca ceremony with the hope of finding clarity. Instead, her journey left her with a strong message to "get her house in order." This confused her at the time, but six months later, when she realized that her emotionally abusive marriage was no longer salvageable, she remembered the message as she was filing for divorce.

In retrospect, she understood that the marriage and the pain it was causing needed to be addressed before she could make any big career decisions.

nothing happened, maybe the medicine is telling you that you're not broken. Sometimes you may have to go where the trip takes you rather than trying to force an outcome. Said differently, you may intend to get to point D, but the medicine needs to bring you to points A, B, and C first.

## Set and Setting: Preparing for Takeoff

It bears repeating: *Set* refers to your mindset—mood, personality, beliefs, and perceptions. *Setting* refers to the environment—the room you're in, the people around you, the music, the smells, the weather, and so on. Psychedelics amplify both lenses, so it's important to be aware of and intentional about both set and setting at the outset of your trip.

### PREPARING YOUR SET

Psychedelic historian Ido Hartogsohn writes that LSD "acts as a mirror and magnifying glass to its user's state of mind." If the mind is anxious, he says, "LSD could easily function as an anxiety inducing drug. If it is creative, then it could equally serve as a creativity enhancer.

Should it be spiritual, then spirituality will be enhanced."[1] Given this mirroring effect, it's essential that you prepare your state of mind—your set—before you trip, because no matter your stated intention, it's likely that the drug will take on, or mirror, your set.

In fact, consider approaching the entire experience as a three-day journey rather than a one-day jaunt:

**Day one, before the trip:**

- Stay quiet and unhurried.
- Make time for self-reflection. Spend part of the day in nature if possible.
- Do a digital detox—steer clear of media and social media that is violent, aggressive, or heavy.
- Reaffirm your intention, and if you're working with a guide, clarify these thoughts or any lingering concerns you might have to create a deeper sense of calm. If you're on your own, open your journal and explore them in writing.
- Eat lightly and refrain from alcohol.

# USING PHOTOS TO SPARK INTENTIONS

Images can trigger emotions that transcend words and a box of photos once helped me clarify my intentions prior to a ketamine journey. I went into the session with no clear focus, yet the photos I selected triggered questions and memories that were lurking just below the surface. The results of that session are still with me today.

Here's how it works:

- Get hold of a box of Magnum postcards (or any postcard box set you like).
- Amble through the collection and select two photos that mean the most to you. Tell your trip partner why these images matter.
  * What do they bring to mind?
  * What memories do they stimulate?
  * What future projection or fantasy do they spark?
- Ask your trip partner to respond to what you're saying by doing reflective listening or sharing what your words bring up for them. If you are on your own, journal your responses or record them.
- Continue expanding the story. Give yourself plenty of time to embellish or go deeper. Then move to the next image.
- Take at least thirty minutes to complete the exercise.

*Note:* If you don't have a box of images, open any art or photography book, or select photos from your own archive. Give yourself a wide selection of people, places, or landscapes to choose from.

- Listen to music, read poetry, or do something uplifting.
- Clean your house. Honestly, a tidy environment that doesn't remind you of all the chores you haven't done is more serene.
- Be gentle with your body, mind, and spirit.

**Day two, the trip.**

**Day three, after the trip:**

- Stay quiet. If you feel a shift in your mindset, create the space and devote the time to let something new come in.
- Expect to feel vulnerable. Welcome it!
- Pay attention to new sensitivities; they may be fleeting. Record your insights.
- Do not make any big decisions or draw conclusions; stay open to what comes up.

### PREPARING YOUR SETTING

Just as your set could have a profound impact on your experience, so, too, could your setting—the location and circumstances that surround you during your trip.

## "Go to the meadows, go to the garden, go to the woods. Open your eyes!"

—ALBERT HOFMANN

## LONG, SLOW PREPARATION

As the psychedelic movement gathers steam, new models of preparation (and integration) are appearing. An increasing number of practitioners I've encountered are blending ancestral practices into their preparation. Often this will begin weeks or months before the journey so that people can build bridges to the "spirit world," or "nagual" as Carlos Casteneda defined it, and to each other. Methods vary depending on which ancestral tradition they derive from and can consist of everything from drum circling to choosing an animal or an ancestor to accompany people in the altered state should things get confusing or difficult. Long preparation also helps people to become more proficient at understanding the deeper layers of their intentions and what they're hoping to get out of the journey. It is said to allow people to journey more deeply because they have made themselves more vulnerable while at the same time tethering them to a community of like-minded others.

### Tripping Indoors

If you're tripping indoors, choose a clean, comfortable space with a couch or bed, along with access to a toilet. You'll likely want to lie down at some point, so make sure there are soft pillows and blankets. Your goal is to create a simple environment that supports inner tranquility,

## YOUR BRAIN ON MUSIC

In addition to the place and the people you're tripping with, music is the third ingredient to ensuring a pleasant or healing, experience. Most Indigenous cultures use some form of music, rhythmic chanting, or drumming to ease the transition from one level of awareness to another and to enhance the feeling of safety through nonverbal support. "Music can regenerate our emotions and heal," says Dr. Frederick Barrett, director of the Center for Psychedelic and Consciousness Research at Johns Hopkins. It can also trigger memories, connect us with our nostalgic selves, and create new neural pathways that lead to positive emotions during sessions. "The entire brain listens to music," Barrett says. "Psychedelics turn the volume up to 11."[2]

Since the late 1960s, therapists have used music to help patients navigate the psychological experience of the trip. One of the most influential voices in this space was Helen Bonny, a music therapist who was hired at the Maryland Psychiatric Research Center in 1968 to work alongside Walter Pahnke, the psychiatrist and minister who led the early Good Friday Experiment.

At the time, therapists were choosing music randomly and on the fly—no one had codified a system to help subjects disconnect from worldly concerns and get lost in the emotional content of the trip without, as Bonny put it, "being burdened by intellectualizations and intellectual reactions." Bonny suggested soothing music for takeoff; driving music during the peak; and calming, familiar music to land. She also advised avoiding music that could spark associations (such as religious or choral music) until the subject was so immersed in the trip that the style of music would not matter.[3]

You of course should feel free to create your own. Music you love or that's particular to your own life experience can be comforting and joyous. I enjoy some of East Forest's soundtracks for takeoff and often prefer to tune in to birds, waves, or the wind as things ramp up. Some people find music with words or discordant sounds distracting. It's a matter of taste. If you are listening to music, closing your eyes or covering them with an eyeshade pillow or cloth will increase its impact. Some people prefer to keep their eyes open. It's your choice.

so consider amenities such as flowers, art, incense, and a sound system, all of which can soothe or stimulate your senses. Steer clear of anything that looks or smells medical/medicinal. It may also be wise to avoid overly loud or frenetic environments such as house parties, bars, or people you don't feel comfortable with.

### Tripping Outdoors

Connecting to grass, trees, birds, water, and sky can make the journey softer and more soothing. If you're outside, make sure you're away from strangers—psychedelics, especially high-dose journeys, can make you super sensitive to the presence of unexpected others. Bring along a blanket and maybe some music and be sure there is a comfortable place to lie down. Of course, many trips combine indoor and outdoor environments.

## GUIDES, TRIPSITTERS, THERAPISTS

There is an ongoing conversation about whether to choose a guide or a therapist or a trusted friend when using psychedelics. No matter which you choose, an ideal trip partner has experience with psychedelics—both taking them and escorting others through a trip. As Dr. Jeffrey Guss, psychiatrist, psychoanalyst, and lead trainer with Fluence, a psychedelic therapy training center, puts it, "The presence of a wise, calm, caring, attuned person is exactly what's needed to allow you to safely and maximally surrender into your journey."* Dr. Guss's checklist for selecting a guide or therapist is as follows:

- Ask people you trust for referrals, and be sure to ask any potential guide for their referrals, too.
- Check their credentials, but don't base your decision solely on this. What's their training? Are they a highly credentialed psychotherapist or an underground practitioner with years of experience? Look for a good fit.
- Is this person clear about fees and the parameters of treatment?
- Listen to what they say beyond their words: Does this person make you feel safe, calm, and eager to explore?
- Can this person tolerate extreme states of emotion in other people without panicking?
- What other work have they done previous to their psychedelic support career? Has this person helped other people? (The answer should be yes.)
- Does this person ask questions that expand your narrative? Does this person relate to you in a way that feels authentic and boundaried, but at the same time warm and caring?
- Does this person seem to like you? Do you like them?
- What does this person's space look like?
- Has this person tamed their own grandiosity and narcissism?
- Does this person's sense of humor align with yours? Humor is very important when tripping!

---

* Some professionals are uncomfortable when asked if they have experience with psychedelics, worried they could lose their license by doing something illegal, but c'mon! As Dr. Guss says, "Would you go to a yoga teacher who had never sat on a mat or a psychoanalyst who had never been on a couch? I'd be sure my practitioner has not only used psychedelics but has benefited from them."

# "The psychedelic space is both saturated and completely open at the same time. There is no protocol for integration."

—DR. IDO COHEN

## SHIFTING OUT OF DARK PLACES

There's a Buddhist saying: "Invite your demon to tea, and see what you learn."

Challenging trips typically occur when something arises that you're trying to resist. Resistance tends to exacerbate difficult moments. Try to welcome the darkness. If you're being chased by a five-hundred-pound bear with paws the size of your head but your guide says, "How wonderful!" it can serve as an invitation to reframe what's going on.

Other useful interventions:

- Hold someone's hand. Sometimes just a gentle touch can redirect your mind.
- Change the music.
- Go outside into nature.
- Hug someone or some pillows.
- Look at photos of people you love, a newborn baby, a garden—something that brings you joy.
- Stare into a flower. James Fadiman calls

such nonverbal interventions "a method of depth psychological work without form, without vocabulary."[4] Flowers make sense to people who are tripping in ways that transcend words.

## Integration: A Smooth Landing

In the days, weeks, or months following psychedelics, you may notice an internal shift or feel more sensitized to the world around you. Integration is the process of surfacing and interacting with feelings, images, and observations that emerged in the non-ordinary state of consciousness. It's the work that ensures that the trip becomes more than just another memory. It is both an active and a passive process that relies on curiosity, exploration, and introspection. Don't think of it as a conclusion: Think of integration as continuing the dialogue that started on the trip. And it doesn't have to be a therapeutic process. It can be playful!

Integration is a nebulous process without guidelines that varies among individuals and cultures. To indigenous peoples, visionary plant medicines are used regularly as a part of daily life. Concepts of mind, body, spirit, medicine, and nature are not viewed as separate entities; they are part of a unified whole. Illness occurs when these elements go out of balance and these peoples use plant medicines to realign the elements and heal. They aren't grounded in intellectual understandings of the world but instead rely on mythical and cultural references that help them make sense of the symbolic and often abstract content that comes up in a trip. Westerners grounded in the scientific tradition don't have these understandings. We view the trip as an experience distinct from everyday reality, so integration or therapeutic support can help us expand our capacity for insight, healing, and perhaps change.

How you integrate pretty much depends on who you journey with, but definitely make time to do it. "After the ecstasy, the laundry," is how renowned meditation teacher Jack Kornfield explains the need to do the hard work following the revelation of any ecstatic insight.

Some people integrate with a therapist. If you're not comfortable medicalizing the mystical, if you have an existing spiritual practice, or if a journey has led you in a more transcendental direction, consider contacting a modern chaplain. Many are interfaith practitioners who hold a more flexible stance on the mysteries of the spirit than traditional chaplains affiliated with organized religions, and they are stepping into psychedelic counseling.*

### INTEGRATION CIRCLES

If you're not working with a practitioner but want to integrate with others, consider joining an integration circle. Some very experienced psychonauts believe that the power of psychedelics lies more in the community interaction following a journey than in the medicine itself.

"Hearing other people's experiences can help you 'de-shame' what you're struggling with," says psychologist Ido Cohen. "When you hear a similar version of your story mentioned by other people, you realize that you're not as bad, or lonely, or odd as you thought you were. Eliminating shame opens up space to get more curious about what happened to you. I think shame is the biggest hurdle to transformation. In our community circles, we talk about 'the

> **"Think of expressive writing as a life course correction as opposed to something you have to commit to doing every day for the rest of your life."**
> —JAMES PENNEBAKER

village model of learning,' which means we're all here to learn from each other."

Some people who get psychedelicized can feel isolated from their friends who aren't doing psychedelics. "So, it feels good to go to a space where you're in the company of people practicing the same things."

### DIY INTEGRATION

Sometimes there's a lag between the experience and the ability to make meaning from it, which is one reason it's useful to have the tools to integrate on your own. Sometimes you want to hold things close before letting them out into the wild. Sometimes there are just no words to describe the ineffable. And sometimes you

---

* The term *chaplain* is sometimes used interchangeably with the term *spiritual care provider* or *spiritual care practitioner*. Chaplains in the US generally have a master's degree in theological education, a year of supervised clinical training, and sometimes ordination. In addition to academic qualifications, chaplains are often endorsed by a religious or spiritual group, which adds another layer of accountability.

may not be able to afford a therapist. Any contemplative practice—meditation, journaling/writing, art, music, smoking your favorite cannabis and lingering with the experience, communing with nature, working with clay, dance, any form of play—can help metabolize your psychedelic experience.

### Journaling

James Pennebaker, research scientist and author of *Opening Up by Writing It Down*, has shown that journaling can work as effectively as talk therapy to heal emotional wounds, lead to a greater sense of well-being, decrease stress, and improve relationships.

### Step 1: Journal for Twenty to Thirty Minutes a Day for Four Days Maximum

To get the most from your journaling, make an appointment with the page at the same time for three or four days in a row. Sit in the same spot—a cozy spot, a spot you like to be in. Switch your phone to airplane mode and face the page. Limit your sessions to twenty to thirty minutes. No more, as overwriting can lead to rumination.

Even if you think you have nothing to write, put your pen (or pencil) on the page and record whatever comes to mind in the moment. Abandon yourself to the process: Words, pictures, doodles, physical sensations. Something. Anything. Everything. Just begin. Capture the details of your journey, however random they may seem, even things that don't mean much to you at this point. Use the first person and present tense to increase recall and avoid analysis. Something like "I close my eyes and see a

swirling rainbow-colored forest that pulses in sync with the singing of a robin." At the very least you'll have a record of harvested observations that will be with you for the rest of your life. Try these probes to jog your curiosity:*

- What, if anything, has shifted?
- What images do you recall?
- Is there something you knew in your head that now feels true in your heart? Some newly revealed truth?
- Were you reminded of anything that you haven't thought about in years?
- Were you able to get out of your old self-narrative? To reframe the story you tell yourself about yourself in a new way?
- What five words best describe your experience?
- What sensations are most alive in your body? Where?
- What parts of yourself did you let go of?
- Were there any parts that died or were reborn?
- What felt most challenging? Most rewarding?
- What was the One Best Thing that happened?

### Step 2: Home In on a Few Essential Themes

Look at what you've written. What feels most alive? Pick three to five themes to prioritize.

### Step 3: Make an Implementation Plan—but Hold It Lightly

What are two or three things you can do going

---

* Thank you, Julia Christina Reibelt, for your great Substack series, *The Journey,* and agreeing to share your thoughts on spiritual and emotional integration as well as intention setting in this book.

forward? This can vary, from seeing more (or less) of certain people, to taking on (or dropping) a new challenge, to starting (or quitting) an exercise or creative routine, to sharing your writing with a therapist or spiritual guide. Some people develop a simple mantra, such as "I'm enough" or "I belong" or "I have purpose," which they then practice throughout the day.

Don't make any obligations, steadfast rules, or big changes at this point. Small steps only and hold them lightly. "An action plan can work great, but very often psychedelics are nonlinear," notes psychedelic chaplain Daan Keiman. "Sometimes a psychedelic is showing you to get out of your comfort zone, and that can't be planned. Strike the right balance between listening to what you need in the moment and sticking to your plan."[5]

## SPIRITUAL INTEGRATION

You don't have to be religious to experience spiritual amplification under a psychedelic. The German word for "God," *Gott*, is derived from the word for "to invoke" or "to call," as in to invite a higher being to join you. Throughout time, even agnostics and atheists have noticed that psychedelics can offer a glimpse of some higher power. "I was struck by a woman who identified as an atheist yet described her psilocybin journey as being 'bathed in God's love,'" said Brian C. Muraresku, the author of *The Immortality Key*. "When asked what an atheist's version of 'God's Love' felt like, she said, 'Probably like your mother's love felt like when you were an infant . . . ' There are very few therapeutic modalities or technologies that can evoke the powerful bond between infant and parent. To me, that qualifies as a spiritual moment."[6]

Try these probes as you think about your spiritual integration:

- What transcendent quality has this journey invoked for you?
- Has anything that was hovering just outside your awareness become clear?
- What paradoxical or nondual understandings did you arrive at? What was Both/And?
- Did any images stand out? What might they signify to you?
- What core beliefs about yourself did you uncover? Which of these feed you or which do you want to let go of?
- Are there any relationships or practices you want to cultivate or relinquish?
- If you do have an existing spiritual or religious practice . . .

   Has your journey led you to renew your commitment to it or has it pointed out things that you need to wrestle with?

   Was it guiding you to more deeply embody your spiritual beliefs? If so, is there a practice, or a community that shares your philosophy that you could become more involved with?

## EMOTIONAL INTEGRATION

Emotions can expand oceanically on psychedelics. Sometimes they are processed during the journey, but other times they barely surface or feel jumbled; you have to let them bubble up before exploring them.

Try these probes as you consider your emotional integration:

- What familiar (or unfamiliar) emotions arose?

- How do you feel about these emotions? Scared? Joyous? Curious?
- Which of your emotion-driven behaviors are avoidant or harmful, and why? Which are useful?
- Are there any conversations you may want to have? How do you feel about those conversations?
- What support can you ask for from family, friends, or professionals? Is asking for support easy or challenging? How can you make it more enjoyable?

## SOMATIC INTEGRATION

Friedrich Nietzsche once said, "There is more wisdom in your body than in your deepest philosophy." Somatic therapy helps you recognize feelings as physical sensations in the body. Somatic integrators use every modality under the sun—acupuncture, cranial osteopathy, breathwork, body scanning—to find where trauma is held and to assist the body to naturally release that emotion. Other approaches, including yoga, qigong, tai chi, flotation tanks, Gaga Dance, or 5Rhythms dance, can help you drop your emotional defenses and open your body-heart-spirit complex. Explore what feels right for you.

## DON'T FORGET ABOUT PLAY!

The more psychedelics come to be seen as treatments for diseases, the greater the risk of misunderstanding them as just another cog in the Western medical model. Psychedelics have always been far more interesting than that. They are, by nature, creative, and have the potential to open us to a more playful or creative approach to life. "We can mistake play for 'fun,'" says Ross Ellenhorn, a psychologist and the author of *Purple Crayons: The Art of Drawing a Life.* "But even though fun is definitely something we do that is playful, play is very serious business when it comes to exploring what occurred in your trip."

In other words, feel free to use integration to explore your newly fertilized imagination. If a psychedelic unleashes the urge to draw, mold clay, sing, debate, try improv theater, make a speech, or do something outside of your comfort zone that liberates you from the seriousness that may be constraining your life, try it. Psychedelics have the ability to loosen not only your thinking but also the boxes with which you conceive of your "self."

## HOW LONG SHOULD I WAIT BEFORE TRIPPING AGAIN?

The rule of thumb is: The more profound the experience, the longer you should wait before going at it again.[7]

If you feel the rush to do psychedelics again immediately following a trip, or without integration, you may be setting yourself up for trouble. There's no set rule about time off between trips, but make sure you've passed through the period of vulnerability and have landed fully back on earth. That can sometimes take weeks, not days. These medicines may not be physically addictive, but you can put yourself in harm's way or allow yourself to be too open to suggestions or bad actors.

# SETTING AN INTENTION OR INTEGRATING CAN BE AS SIMPLE AS A WALK IN THE WOODS

## BY ROBERT BRAY

(Bray is certified as a forest therapy guide by the Association of Nature and Forest Therapy Guides and Programs, whose resources have inspired and are quoted in this piece.)

Forest bathing is a gentle amble through nature, usually guided, that allows participants to slow down and attune their senses to what the natural world is presenting. It's not a hike, you don't walk too far, and there is no destination. Forest (or desert or beach) bathing promotes the well-being of both people and the land through guided immersions in the environment. It can activate memories, senses, and emotions to support health and happiness.

Inspired by *shinrin-yoku* (Japanese for "forest bathing"), the practice was origin-ally conceived in the 1980s as Japan was experiencing dramatic technological and industrial change.

Dr. Qing Li, one of the foremost experts in forest medicine, describes a DIY version of *shinrin-yoku* in a park: "Leave behind your phone, camera, music, and any other distraction. Leave behind your expectations. Slow down; forget about time. Come into the present moment. Find a spot to sit—on the grass, beside a tree, or on a park bench. Notice what you hear and see. Notice what you feel." Japanese researchers have shown that this simple activity of being aware of your awareness lowers pulse rates, increases vigor, and reduces depression, fatigue, and anxiety.

Forest therapy is loosely structured by a sequence of "invitations" designed to allow the participant's senses to open. Breathe in the terpenes and phytoncides, or protective "essential oils" of trees and plants; feel the tingle on your skin in a forest hung with mist; taste the air, a wet stone, or tart pine tips; tune in to the gentle waters of a nearby creek; savor the scent of wet fallen leaves.

These slow walks in nature are constructed to allow participants to spend time in silence, observing with a quiet and accepting presence and reconnecting with their senses and their innate creative potential.

In his useful and inspiring pocket guide *Healing Trees,* Ben Page, a leader in the Association of Nature and Forest Therapy, describes what can happen when you pay attention to nature. "You might notice that you are also remembering how to experience the world through what is called the imaginal sense, of the inner knowing of the heart. The imaginal can be described as a reverie or daydream that comes over us when we slow down our thinking minds. These dreams do not originate within us but instead move through us, connecting us to what is mysterious and unexplainable."

Consider forest bathing as part of your intention setting or integration practice. You can find a local certified forest therapy guide at anft.earth or use the invitations below to practice on your own.

### INVITATIONS

**Sit Spot:** Find a comfortable space—under a tree, against a rock, on a bench—and sit there for fifteen or twenty minutes. The longer you sit, the more you notice. Let things around you reveal themselves when they choose. Invite patience, curiosity, imagination, sensuousness, and playfulness to sit with you. Notice what unfolds around and within you.

**The Joy of Tiny Things:** As you wander through the forest, notice small things on the ground. Which of them captivate you? What is their relationship to other beings, large and small? Notice what you are noticing.

**Green Palaces:** Slowly wander through a forest as if you were touring a grand house. Notice when you cross invisible boundaries between one space and the next—a shift in light, a new smell, or a vibe that becomes more vivid. Wonder how these sensory experiences might define a portal into a new "room" in your green palace. Does that room have a name? Observe what changes as you move through portals and rooms.

**The Gesture of Textures:** Touch the bark of a tree or the smoothness of a rock or the fuzziness of moss. Can some of these textures be safely tasted and do they have a scent? Collect a few textures, tastes, and scents, and if you are walking with someone, share something about the texture of your being.

**Eye Cloud:** Find a place to lie down and gaze up at the sky. Notice the clouds and their movement and shifting patterns. Take time to give your attention to other beings or objects above you—a bird, a leaf, a swaying branch, even your gently waving hand. What are you noticing?

**Symphony of Cedars:** Pick any tree that calls to you and sit under it. Listen to the sounds you hear in and around this tree, from the top branches and canopy down to the trunk and roots. What sounds are so soft, you must get close to hear them? How do all the noises of this forest, including your tree and your body, cocreate a symphony?

**Heart Radar:** Stand comfortably, place your hands over your heart, and take three deep breaths. Pause. Now, orienting your attention to your heart, with your eyes gently closed or softly open, slowly rotate your body in a circle. Notice if your heart is pulling you in any direction. Stop moving, open your eyes, and wander off in the direction felt by your heart, allowing your heart to guide you. What is calling you there? Do they have a scent? Collect a few textures, tastes, and scents, and if you are walking with someone, share something about the texture of your being.

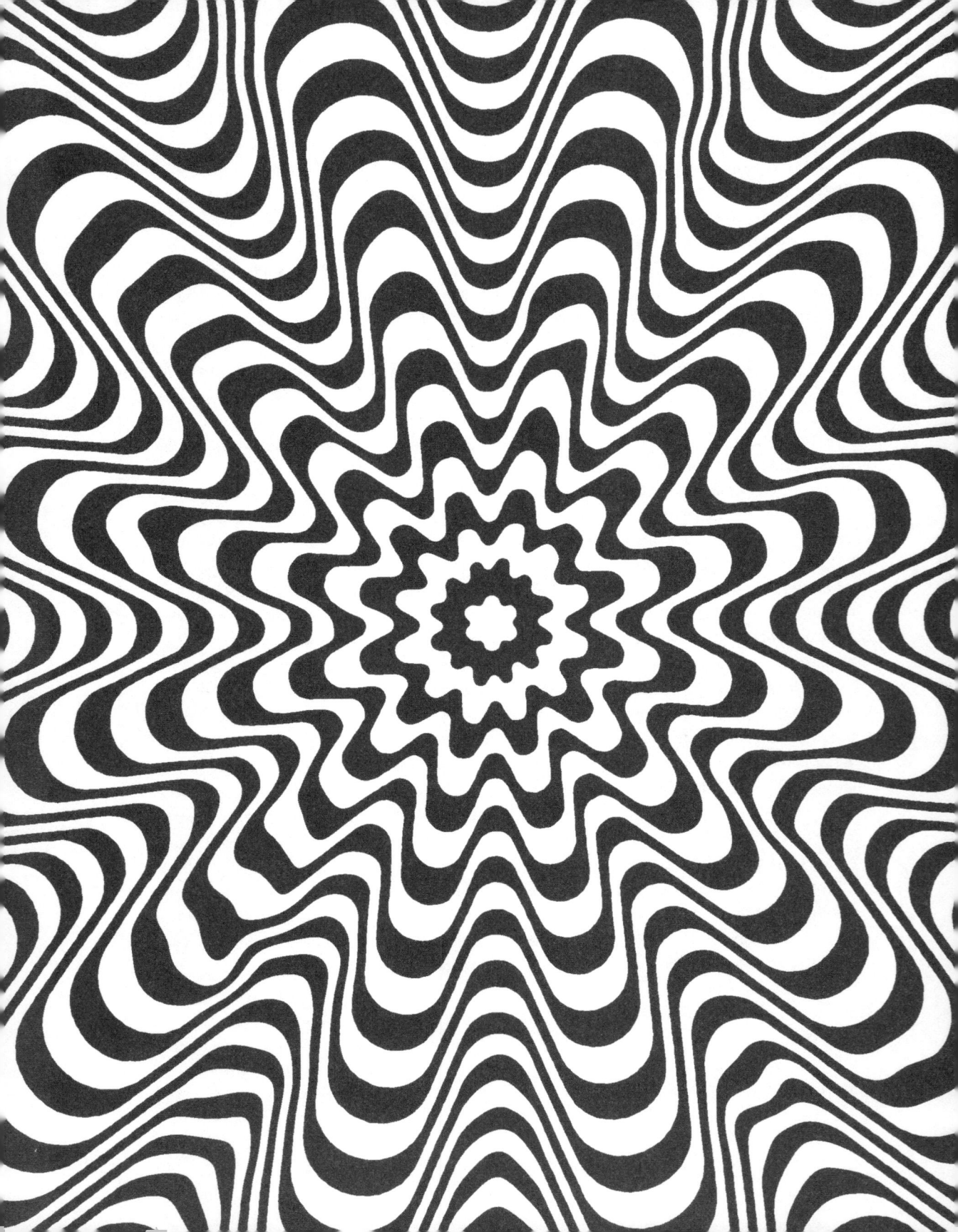

# THE
# SUBSTANCES

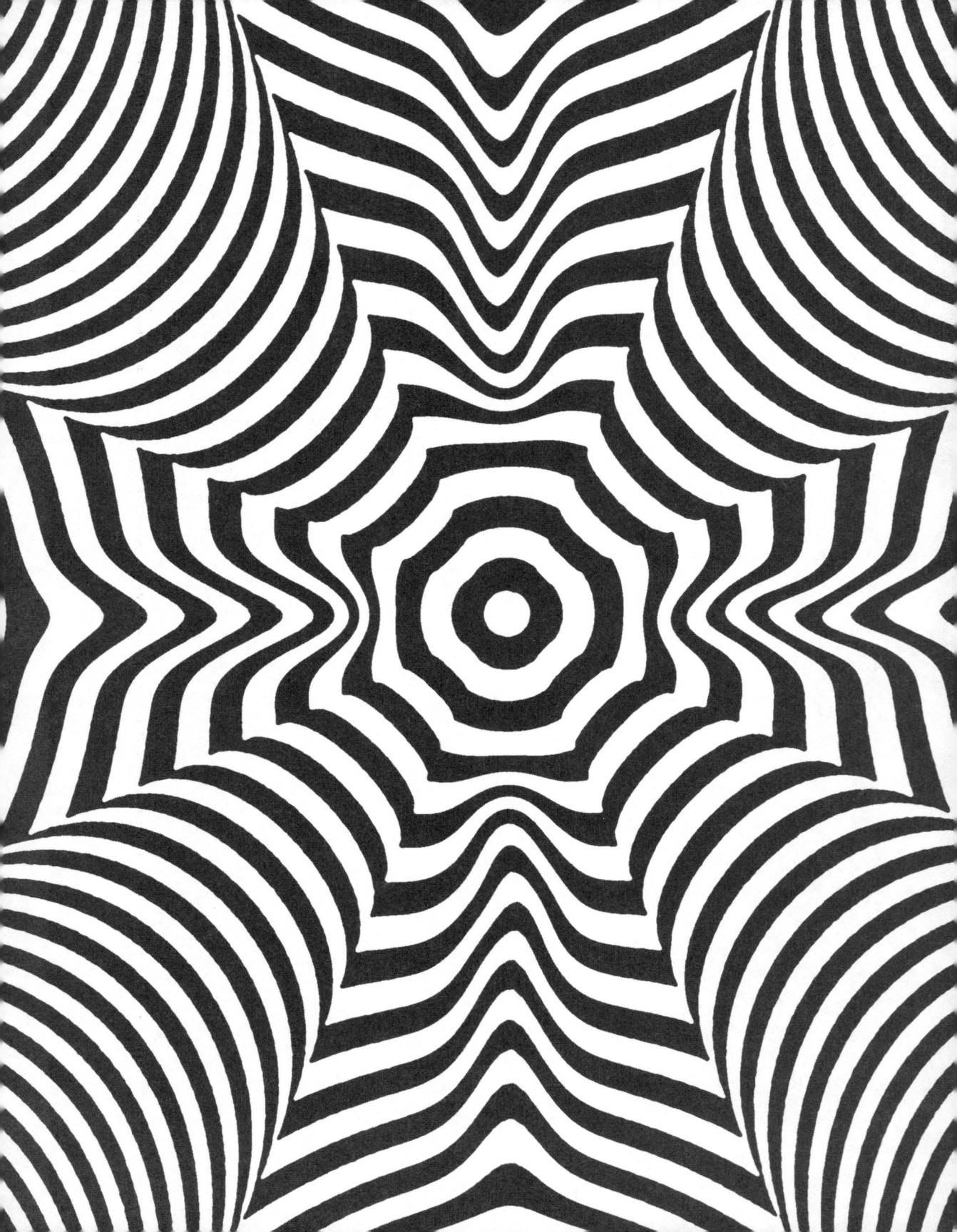

# THE SUBSTANCES*

---

* The dosing guidelines in the following section are reliable parameters to help you design the experience you desire. They have been determined by a synthesis of reliable sources and scientific studies over decades. These include clinical trials, pharmaceutical studies, and, in many cases, the detailed and time-tested formulas of Alexander Shulgin, which underground chemists have relied on for over thirty-five years. I have cross-referenced scientific guidelines with the thousands of contributions and hacks from citizen scientists found in the Erowid vaults and ICEERS (the International Center for Ethnobotanical Education, Research, and Service) and PsychonautWiki libraries.

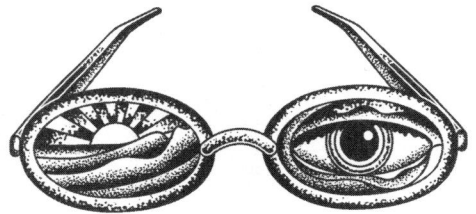

# MDMA

## THE FEELING OPTIMIZER FOR THE OPTIMAL FEELING: LOVE*

------------------------------------------------------------------------

There is nothing but pure euphoria. I have never felt so great or believed this to be possible ... I felt like a citizen of the universe rather than a citizen of the planet ... I have lived all my life to get here ... I have come home. I am complete.[1]

ALEXANDER SHULGIN, *PiHKAL*

Scientists don't use the word *love*; they find it more acceptable to talk about "positive subjective effects." But when you combine empathy, forgiveness, and connection ... well ... love is what you get. MDMA enables an openhearted emotional communion, a sense of trust and forgiveness for others and, importantly, for yourself. It increases tactility: Someone's finger grazing your arm can cause you to feel the rising of every hair. MDMA also builds a powerful connection with nature and the arts, particularly music. In some cases, aftereffects may linger—studies from the UK show that people at raves are able to regenerate the feelings of joy for weeks after a journey.

Compared with other psychedelics MDMA evokes a gentler, subtler, more controllable experience that invites, rather than compels, intense feelings and self-exploration.[2]

The more spiritually inclined have compared it to advanced meditation. One renegade Zen teacher** said, "Ecstasy [MDMA] is a wonderful tool for teaching. I had a student who never succeeded in meditation until Ecstasy removed the block." A Benedictine monk said that the drug facilitated the "awakened attitude all monks seek."[3]

**Also known as:** Molly, Ecstasy, X, XTC, E, the love drug, the hug drug, Mellow Drug of America, ADAM.

**Source:** Synthetic.

**Chemical name:** 3,4-methylenedioxy-N-methylamphetamine.

**Drug classification:** Empathogen; entactogen; stimulant; phenethylamine; amphetamine. Confusingly, while MDMA is classified as an amphetamine, it does not contain amphetamine, the molecule. Translation: It is speedy but it is not speed.

**Methods of administration:** Oral.

**Duration:** 3–6 hours.

**Open critical period:** 3 weeks.

------------------------------------------------------------------------

\* This epigram is based on a quote from Claudio Naranjo, the Chilean psychiatrist, author, and pioneer of integrating Eastern spiritual traditions into Western psychotherapy.

\*\* It's unusual for strict Buddhists to dabble with or encourage substance use.

## RISKS AND ADVERSE EFFECTS

Side effects have been reported by users and include:

- Elevated blood pressure, pulse rate, and temperature
- Dilated pupils
- Diminished appetite
- Jaw clenching and teeth grinding
- Dry mouth
- Dizziness
- Headache
- Nausea
- Eye twitching (nystagmus)
- Tiredness and depressed mood, possibly for days following the journey
- One other less noted side effect is short-term immunosuppression.[4]

## ONE COMPOUND, MANY NAMES

When it debuted in the 1970s, the letters in MDMA were scrambled and it was called Adam. Some therapists said it returned users to a more innocent state, as in the Garden of Eden—that was a bit of a stretch.

When it hit the club scene, it was christened Empathy and/or Therapy, until suppliers realized that no one wanted to go to a club for therapy.

It was rebranded Ecstasy, but after years of tainted samples and the ensuing negative publicity, suppliers rechristened it molly, which is short for "molecule." They thought this term would indicate a purer version of MDMA.

- Deaths from pure MDMA are rare; most MDMA-implicated deaths are the result of a dose tainted with fentanyl, methamphetamine, or another contaminant.
- Overheating: MDMA increases core body temperature, which increases the risks of overheating. This is compounded by being in a hot environment (like a crowded club), heavy physical exertion, taking too large a dose, or mixing with other temperature-raising drugs like cocaine or speed.
- Dehydration and overhydration: Drinking too much or too little water on MDMA can be dangerous due to hypernatremia (dehydration) or hyponatremia (overhydration). The remedy is to drink water steadily without overhydrating. If you're dancing, sip your trip. Take a sip (not a gulp) of water every other song.[5]
- Severe headache: Pounding headaches on any stimulant may be a sign of dangerously high blood pressure. Seek medical attention for a splitting headache that doesn't quit.
- Hypertension, tachycardia, arrhythmia: There is a lot of contradictory information when it comes to MDMA and heart conditions. If you have high blood pressure or arrhythmia or if you're obese, occasional use can strain the cardiovascular system. If you're healthy, a moderate dose of MDMA should not strain your heart. However, if you're using MDMA on a weekly or more frequent basis, a) it's a bad idea, and b) studies show that you may develop valvular heart disease.

- MDMA and SSRIs: It's commonly believed that combining SSRIs with MDMA is dangerous, but it's more likely that SSRIs will blunt or cancel out the effects of MDMA and you'll end up taking too much. According to Dr. Ben Sessa, "At raves, you see people walking around saying that the MDMA didn't work. When we ask if they're on Prozac [or another SSRI], they almost always say 'Yes!'"

- Addiction and overuse: Most research concurs that MDMA does not cause physical dependence, but it can take on too great an importance in people's lives, which results in compulsive use. Get help if you're using it every weekend!

- Tolerance: Occurs after a week of steady use. A seven-day drug holiday typically reverses tolerance.

### More Use, Less Magic

It's wise to limit use to once every three to six months for three reasons:

1. Users report that repeated doses do not extend or increase the empathogenic effects but that the unpleasant "amphetamine-like" side effects become more pronounced with more frequent use.

2. MDMA may become more harmful with frequent and excessive use.'[6] While it's generally safe in moderate doses, the risk of long-term damage to the heart and the brain's serotonin system increases if you roll every weekend.

3. The more you take, the less magic you feel over time. *This is important.* Repeated administrations create a cumulative tolerance, regardless of the amount of time that elapses between doses.

### CONDITIONS ADDRESSED

PTSD, depression, phobias, alcohol use disorder (AUD), alexithymia (inability to describe one's emotions). Before MDMA was prohibited, it was used in couples and group therapy with positive results.

### DOSING GUIDELINES
#### Low dose: 20–80 mg

Low doses are not recommended for most. They can cause physical stimulation and anxiety or discomfort without euphoria or enhanced sociability.

#### Average dose: 80–120 mg

Peak effects for most people occur at around 90 mg.[7]

#### High dose: 120–150 mg

Positive effects begin to drop off in this range, while unpleasant physical effects become much more present. An upper limit for MDMA is 150 to 200 mg. Over 200 mg can be unpleasant and harmful.

---

* The neurotoxicity of MDMA after repeated use is hotly debated. While it was once thought that even a single, moderate dose of MDMA could cause long-term brain damage, new research paints a different picture: Following twelve months of abstinence, chronic users have been shown not to have sustained lasting neural damage. Some studies suggest that while MDMA itself is not neurotoxic, its metabolites may be. Neurotoxicity in humans can be hard to study because many MDMA users also use other drugs, so the long-term effects cannot be solely attributed to one substance.

## MORE IS NOT MORE!

Unlike other drugs, MDMA's desired effects don't have a linear spectrum of intensity. In other words, more MDMA does not necessarily equal more euphoria. The optimal dose sits within a relatively narrow range. Low doses are insufficient to "break through," and high doses incur more side effects with diminishing returns on positive effects. Some people report taking another half dose (40 mg or 60 mg) as a booster 90 to 120 minutes into a session. This can extend the effects for an additional hour or two but only modestly exacerbates speedy side effects such as teeth clenching or eye twitching.

## IS IT SAFE TO USE VIAGRA WITH MDMA?

It's a good question and one that's frequently asked considering that about 40 percent of men say they can't get hard or ejaculate when on MDMA.[8] "From a pharmacological point of view, we just do not see any significant interactions between the two drugs," says Dr. Ben Sessa. The amphetamine effects of MDMA constrict blood flow, whereas Viagra/Cialis dilates arteries and veins, so the two drugs are not acting synergistically, which is a good thing. Also, MDMA acts on the brain, whereas drugs like Viagra or Cialis act peripherally on smooth muscles.

### PROGRESSION OF A TYPICAL JOURNEY

**Liftoff:** Thirty to forty-five minutes. First comes a smile—all is well with the outer and inner world—then a warm cascade of euphoria.

**Peak:** One and a half to two hours. An expansive sense of connection to your inner self, the people you're with, the universe. You may begin to sweat, but you'll love every drop.

**Comedown and landing:** After two hours, the high peaks and you'll be rolling in waves of unconditional love that land you in a soft puddle of tired warmth. Your jaw may be tight from clenching, and you may have a headache, but it's likely the benefits outweigh these effects.

### "Blue Monday" (aka the Ecstasy Crash)

Most users of MDMA are familiar with the post-roll low that follows a journey. For some, it can be a heaviness and lethargy; others experience the crash as a full-on depression that can last for a few days. While some blame the crash on mixing MDMA with other substances or alcohol or dancing nonstop for eight hours, even biochemist Sasha Shulgin, who masterminded his own MDMA and who was not partying at raves, noted the post-roll doldrums.

There are a few steps that might mitigate the symptoms, but none are confirmed by research, so no promises.

1.  Plan two days to trip.

    One for the journey and at least another day for recovery, where you stay quiet, hydrate, eat well, and avoid caffeine.

2.  Reduce the oxidants.

    Dr. Erica Zelfand, a functional medicine physician, psychedelic educator, and CEO of the Right to Heal Clinic in Portland, Oregon, suggests alpha lipoic acid (ALA) supplementation to fight oxidative stress:

    *   300 mg of ALA* at the same time as MDMA, followed by 100 to 150 mg of ALA every one to two hours for the duration of the trip. Conservative practitioners suggest a maximum ALA dose of 2,400 mg in a twenty-four-hour period.
    *   500 to 1,000 mg of vitamin C every two hours the day of the MDMA session. Vitamin C is a great antioxidant; it can also help curb the hyperthermia that comes with MDMA. Use sodium ascorbate, as it's less likely to cause an upset stomach.
    *   Magnesium gluconate: Many people take 330 to 500 mg just before, during, or after MDMA, to minimize jaw clenching and grinding.
    *   5-HTP: Many people use this naturally occurring amino acid and chemical precursor of serotonin, but there's no proof that it works. Try 100 to 400 mg a week before you roll, and wait at least twenty-four hours after you roll to start it again for another two weeks. Note: Do not take 5-HTP immediately after your roll, as it can increase your chances of getting serotonin syndrome. This can make you feel like you have a flu or, if severe, land you in a coma.
    *   P5P: Some people are exploring P5P, a vitamin $B_6$ metabolite that suppresses prolactin and may buffer the crash, but there is no evidence of efficacy. Dr. Andrew Huberman suspects the crash may have less to do with serotonin depletion and more to do with the significant release of dopamine caused by MDMA. "Anytime there's a release of dopamine, there is also a big release of prolactin, a hormone involved in lots of different functions and associated with lethargy." P5P may suppress prolactin and mitigate the crash effects.[9]

3.  Caffeine abstinence.

    It's best to avoid caffeine (including Red Bull and all "energy drinks") on the days before, during, and after MDMA. Caffeine might increase the negative effects of MDMA.

4.  Stick with aspirin.

    If you have a headache, avoid acetaminophen (that's Tylenol in the US, paracetamol in other countries), as it depletes the body's store of an important antioxidant known as glutathione.

---

* Studies indicate that ALA has neuroprotective qualities (as you'd expect of an antioxidant, since neurotoxicity from MDMA use is thought to be caused in large part due to oxidative stress).

## HISTORY

In 1912, Merck synthesized MDMA as a compound to help control bleeding, but it was deemed ineffective. It went unnoticed until Shulgin resynthesized it in 1976. He and his wife, Ann, shared it with Leo Zeff, a psychotherapist who had been using psychedelics therapeutically since 1961.[10] Zeff was on the verge of retiring, but MDMA convinced him to change course. Over the next eight years, he trained about 150 mostly West Coast therapists in MDMA-assisted therapy; collectively they administered an estimated half million doses to some four thousand patients, primarily to couples seeking therapy or to alleviate trauma. Many reported breakthroughs for conditions including depression, phobias, alexithymia (inability to describe one's emotions), and PTSD.[11]

Therapists were nervous about the government banning MDMA so they kept mum about it, but by the early 1980s word was out. Pressed into colorful pills that resembled SweeTarts, MDMA was an instant hit in the world's busiest nightclubs. A group of investors in Texas led by an ex-priest turned yoga/tennis instructor smelled the profit potential of the "love drug" and funded a huge uptick in production and distribution. They even offered free shipping and an 800 number to make ordering easier.[12]

From the dance floors of Studio 54 and The Saint in New York City, MDMA made its way to Ibiza and eventually to warehouse raves in the UK, Berlin, and Amsterdam. The music was acid house; the rhythm was 120 beats per minute, exactly the same as a fetal heart rate and as the drumming that South American shamans used to lift people into a trance state; and the impact was immediate. Raves are one of the few communal ecstatic rituals in Western culture, and they are also hugely profitable: The EDM scene today generates $8.2 billion yearly and is projected to hit $17.5 billion annually by 2031.[13]

The DEA outlawed MDMA in 1985. Scientists and therapists fought in court for three years to make it Schedule 3 so they could continue using it therapeutically, but in 1988 the DEA succeeded in placing it into Schedule 1.

Unsurprisingly, increased public awareness during the scheduling fight produced a surge in use and availability.*

### The Long Road to Legitimization

Once the drug was banned, the number of mental health professionals quietly providing MDMA-assisted therapy dwindled,**[14] as did the numbers of scientists investigating it. But Rick Doblin saw research as the only route to legitimization, and he just wouldn't let it go.

Doblin first encountered MDMA in 1982 at the Esalen Institute in Big Sur, California. (Esalen was the birthplace of the human potential movement.) "Adam" was all the buzz at the time, but Doblin was unimpressed. "It just looked like people were talking to each other. If you can have a conversation on this drug, how important can it be?"[15] But then he tried it, and two years later he formed MAPS, with the Sisyphean (insane?) intent of winning FDA approval for the therapeutic use of MDMA. "Previously I had only thought of myself as a counterculture drug-using

---

* A few hundred thousand people were estimated to use it before prohibition. One recent National Institute on Drug Abuse (NIDA) survey said that 2.2 million Americans used it in 2021. I have no proof, but this estimate strikes me as ridiculously low.

** Torsten Passie, a psychiatrist and drug historian, estimates that sixty thousand patients may have received underground MDMA therapy in the period from 1985 to 2017.

criminal," he told *Playboy*.[16] "But this was my movement into the mainstream. The American legal system allows nonprofit organizations to exist, and you can use them to fight the government." Which is exactly what he did.

It seemed like a pipe dream given the "Just Say No!" antidrug fervor of the Reagan era, but after two decades of fending off alarmist claims about MDMA's supposed dangers, MAPS funded the first clinical trials to treat veterans with PTSD. Results since then have repeatedly exceeded expectations. In 2010 clinical trials run by Michael Mithoefer, MD, and his wife, Annie, just two sessions resolved 83 percent of subjects' PTSD symptoms, no further treatment required.[17]

In 2017 the FDA granted MDMA "breakthrough therapy" status to treat PTSD.[18] After nearly thirty-five years, MDMA was on track to become the first legal psychedelic to treat a medical condition in the US until August 2024, when the FDA criticized the quality of the trials and pretty much quashed chances of approval any time soon.*

## MDMA: A Unicorn among Medicines

The chemical structure of MDMA is related to both amphetamines and mescaline, but its effects are so unique that it is categorized as an empathogen (causing empathy) or an entactogen (from the Greek, "to touch within").

MDMA dumps a chemical cocktail of serotonin and dopamine into the brain, which causes a surge of alertness, motivation, and energy without irritation. Typically, when dopamine drops back to its normal level, you feel irritable and hungry for more, which is what occurs with cocaine or meth. What makes MDMA a unicorn are the massive cascades of serotonin it releases into synapses while it is active in the system. This makes people (and other animals, even grumpy octopuses) more socially connected.

---

## MDMA VERSUS MDA: WHAT'S THE DIFFERENCE?

MDA, methylenedioxy-amphetamine, was synthesized in the 1960s and banned in 1970 before MDMA hit the scene. It is still available on the gray market, but it works and feels different from MDMA.

- MDA is a molecular hybrid between amphetamine and mescaline. It's speedier, it takes longer to hit, and its effects last longer—six to eight hours.
- MDA works more as an empathogen at low doses and more as a psychedelic at high doses.
- MDA reputedly doesn't cause erection difficulties in men.
- MDA is more toxic. Studies from the 1970s showed that it produced some medical complications and even deaths.
- Some people make their MDMA "more psychedelic" by mixing one part MDA to four parts MDMA.

---

* MDMA- and psilocybin-assisted therapies were legalized for medical use in Australia in 2023.

Oxytocin also gets a big boost.[19] The so-called cuddle chemical increases the warm feelings involved in bonding between friends, lovers, parents, kids, and pets. It also increases the pain of breaking those bonds. Net-net: MDMA creates a deeper sense of feeling *everything*.

## MDMA ALSO MINIMIZES FEAR

Psychedelics like psilocybin or LSD tickle the serotonin 2A receptor that is thought to play a role in creating introspective and mystical experiences.

But MDMA is more mood enhancing than mystical. That's because it is also thought to activate the serotonin 1B receptor, which turns on brain functions involved in our desire to socially engage, trust, and discuss anything, positive and negative. "It creates more of an affiliation, a friendliness of sorts, with negative thoughts or feelings, so that they are more easily embraced," says Dr. Andrew Huberman.[20] This "prosocial" effect is verified by research showing that when people on MDMA view photos of scary faces, they see them as less fearsome. They view happy faces more positively, too.[21]

Brain imaging studies show that MDMA calms the connection between two brain areas that affect how we view our inner experience: the amygdala and insula.[22] The amygdala controls many responses, among them fear. The insula maintains balance between our introspective self and the environment.

It's theorized that people with PTSD have a heightened threat detection center in the amygdala-insula circuit, which turns up the volume on agitation when it's triggered. MDMA diminishes this response; in its place, love and forgiveness arise. This allows the door on difficult memories or feelings that is normally slammed shut to open.

"That's a very unique pharmacological effect," says Dr. Ben Sessa. "Many drugs inhibit the fear response—heroin and vodka for example—but they are messy. MDMA is unique pharmacologically. It selectively turns off the fear response but leaves the other faculties intact."

## MORE TRUST, LESS TRAUMA

This is one explanation of how MDMA helps treat severe trauma caused by a sexual assault, violent crime, or war. These capital-T traumas lock in all sorts of maladaptive responses—anxiety, disrupted sleep, fear, social withdrawal—that get triggered in stressful situations. MDMA allows people to examine their own thought patterns with more equanimity and then change how they respond. In popular lingo, it rewires brain circuitry for the long term, often in one dose.

"You see this on patients' faces," says Sessa, "You see this look of, 'Oh my God, maybe I'm not a useless, worthless piece of crap. Maybe there's another story,' and there's an epiphany where they truly believe they're not awful or a piece of crap. That is the crucial experiential component that MDMA and psychedelics give."

## FUTURE APPLICATIONS

Alcohol use disorder (AUD): Alcohol is the legal palliative most widely used to blunt the pain of trauma. Data from a Phase III clinical trial for PTSD shows that MDMA-assisted therapy led to decreased alcohol consumption and decreased hazardous use for individuals with mild AUD.[23] A preliminary study in the UK has shown that MDMA-assisted therapy is safe for patients with AUD, clearing the way for a full study.[24]

Social anxiety and autism spectrum disorder (ASD): For years, people with ASD have

> # "I've studied yoga, it turned out very well. I've studied EMDR, I've started theater groups, I studied neurofeedback, I studied various psychiatric medications. But what we see with MDMA-assisted therapy is really more profound than anything else we have done."
>
> —BESSEL VAN DER KOLK, MD, author of *The Body Keeps the Score*

been using street MDMA because it lowers their social anxiety, enabling them to be calmer, maintain eye contact, and communicate more easily. A pilot study for MDMA-assisted therapy found "rapid and durable improvement" in ASD symptoms.[25] This is hopeful, as standard approaches have limited effectiveness.

Chronic pain: Dr. Andrew Weil has suggested that the relaxed state MDMA induces can help people with chronic pain. "A major component of pain is the subjective experience," he has said.[26] "MDMA changes your perspective about what is going on in your body so it can help people develop a new relationship with chronic pain in which it is less of a discomfort." One small 2022 study noted significant reductions of chronic pain among people with PTSD after MDMA treatment.[27]

Insight and self-awareness: In the 1980s, therapists including Ann Shulgin, Ralph Metzner, and his partner Padma Catell had good

therapuetic results combining MDMA with the mescaline derivative 2C-B to increase patient insights—but no further studies have been conducted. Contraindications included severe heart disease, high blood pressure, history of psychosis, diabetes, epilepsy, and pregnancy.[28]

## MYTHS AND MYTHCONCEPTIONS ABOUT MDMA

### A Single Dose of MDMA Is Dangerously Neurotoxic

In 2002, one of the top scientific journals, *Science*, published a study by George A. Ricaurte claiming that MDMA caused severe neurotoxicity in primates. Since primate brains closely resemble human brains, a predictable media firestorm ensued. The following year, the authors retracted the study, claiming that the primates were "accidentally" injected with the far more toxic methamphetamine (crystal meth, not MDMA). Even though the study was hogwash, the negative publicity persisted.

### MDMA Eats Holes in the Brain

A few years later, Ricaurte struck again with another study claiming that MDMA left holes in people's brains. That, too, was debunked, but not before the media feasted on the headlines. "It's hard to trust George," Dr. Julie Holland, a professor of psychiatry at New York University and editor of *Ecstasy: A Complete Guide*, told *The New York Times*.[29] "He plays games with his data to win more federal grants by making the drugs look bad."

### It Turns Users into Sex Fiends

Unfounded and laughable, especially for men. MDMA heightens sensory awareness and touch, but it impedes erections and (male) orgasm. There's no data on women's orgasms. However, people on MDMA may be more open to sexual overtures, so be sure to discuss consent before tripping.

### Excess Use Causes Cognitive Decline

This is difficult to determine, since most people who use MDMA use other substances as well. A fascinating 2011 study[30] from Harvard looked at a group of Latter-day Saints (Mormons) who had never used caffeine, alcohol, or other substances but who had taken Ecstasy anywhere from 50 to 450 times(!). (The LDS church was obviously late to ban MDMA.) The study found no evidence of decreased cognitive performance.

---

It may be possible to make some assumptions about the purity of your MDMA crystals based on their color. The purest crystals are white and clear. Light brown or light gray crystals probably have a small amount of leftover processing agents in them, but they are generally safe to consume. If your crystals are dark brown, the synthesis was not successful. Chances are, the crystals are not safe and should not be consumed without testing. If they are purple or pink, they may contain added food dye as a marketing ploy, but that is not any indication of purity. Of course, the most certain way to determine purity is through testing (more on this in chapter 7, "Harm Reduction").

---

# MAGIC MUSHROOMS (PSILOCYBIN/PSILOCIN)

## THE FLESH OF THE GODS

------------------------------------------

The problem with psilocybin is that it sounds too good to be true.
We've all been trained that if it sounds too good to be true, it is.
But we've also been trained that there are exceptions to every rule.

PAUL STAMETS, *American mycologist*

**M**agic mushroom is the encompassing term for any species of fungi with psychoactive effects. Of the 14,000 identified strains of mushrooms, 220 are psychedelic[*] and they are found on every continent except Antarctica.[1] Magic mushrooms contain two psychoactive alkaloids—psilocybin and psilocin. Psilocybin is not itself psychoactive—it is rapidly converted to psilocin after ingestion. These alkaloids interact with the serotonin receptors (5-HT2A), producing changes in the way we perceive sensory information, sound, vision, and touch.

Magic mushrooms are also tools for self and spiritual discovery. They have been used in ceremonies and as sacraments in virtually every region of the world in which they are found.

**Also known as:** Shrooms, mushies, *hongos, niños santos.*

**Active ingredients:** Psilocybin, psilocin.
**Chemical names:** Psilocybin: 4-phosphoryloxy-N, N-dimethyltryptamine. Psilocin: 4-hydroxy-N, N-dimethyltryptamine.

**Drug classification:** Serotonergic hallucinogen; tryptamine. Categorized alongside other classical psychedelics such as DMT, LSD, and mescaline.

**Methods of administration:** Oral ingestion (raw or dried), tea, honey, capsules.

**Duration:** 4–6 hours.

**Open critical period:** ~3 weeks.

### RISKS AND SIDE EFFECTS

The risk of physical harm from magic mushrooms is exceptionally low. There has never been a reported death from overdose. Some unwanted side effects can occur. Most are short-term and resolve once the journey ends.

---

[*] Interestingly 1–2 percent of all mushrooms are edible, 1–2 percent are poisonous, and 1–2 percent are psychedelic. The vast majority of mushrooms will neither kill you nor thrill you.

Side effects may include:

- Anxiety and paranoia
- Dilated pupils
- Fatigue or drowsiness
- Headaches
- Slightly increased heart rate and blood pressure
- Lack of coordination
- Muscle weakness
- Nausea and stomach discomfort

## CONDITIONS ADDRESSED

Treatment-resistant depression; end-of-life anxiety; obsessive-compulsive disorder; PTSD; addiction to tobacco, nicotine, and alcohol; cluster headaches and migraines; small-t traumas; increase in positive mood.

## DOSING GUIDELINES

### Microdose: 0.2–0.5 g

A microdose can offer increased focus and concentration, creative generation, and heightened emotionality. It may at first cause slight changes in mood (more social or antisocial), mild euphoria, and alterations in workflow or focus. After one or two weeks, these subtle changes disappear.

### Gentle journey: 0.5–1.5 g

This dose may make everything feel a bit "sparkly"; it may cause a tingly sensation in your stomach or an uptick in mood. Your vision may have slight wavy vibrations, and your hearing could be more sensitive.

Gentle doses are sometimes used to expand creative processes, making you more receptive to new ideas without interfering with linear thinking.

### Power trip: 2–4 g

"Colors are brighter, the world jiggles a bit with energy . . . some cherished beliefs will be disassembled to enable you to judge what's valuable or not . . . a notch up in value for the words 'kindness,' 'closeness' and 'connection.'"
—James Fadiman[2]

### Heroic dose: 5 g+

A heroic dose offers all of the above plus powerful perceptual and somatic effects. Challenging trips are more common at high doses, especially if you're unprepared. Effects will last slightly longer, around six or seven hours. If you're new to psychedelics, consider tripping at this dose with a guide or people you love close by.

*Note:* Psilocybin content varies among mushroom species, which makes precise dosing more challenging than with synthesized compounds. Also, different varieties of mushrooms are known to be more potent than others. The best way to determine the potency of your mushrooms is with a QTest, which you can learn more about in chapter 7.

## DOSING FRESH MUSHROOMS

Fresh mushrooms contain ten times as much water as dry mushrooms, so you will need to multiply your favorite dry dose by ten. For example, the standard 3 g dose of dry mushrooms is equivalent to about 30 g of fresh.

# STAVING OFF NAUSEA

One of the less pleasant side effects of chewing magic mushrooms is nausea. The following preparations may help to reduce this unwanted feeling.

**Lemon Tek**

- Grind dried mushrooms as fine as possible in a portable electric coffee grinder. It will take less than a minute for your mill to pulse the mushrooms into a fine powder.
- Do not open the grinder for at least half an hour. Lifting the lid right away will cause the particles to be sucked up into the air and anoint your kitchen with a fine layer of mushroom fairy dust. Another option: Turn the grinder over and let mushroom dust settle before opening.
- Transfer the ground mushroom powder to a bowl and cover with the juice of one or two lemons—enough to submerge the mushroom powder.
- Marinate for fifteen minutes.
- Drink the mixture or mix it into a smoothie of blended frozen fresh fruits.

**Why it works:** Chitin is the culprit here. It's the natural defense the psilocybin mushroom produces to keep predators away, and it can make you feel queasy.

Powdering dried mushrooms is akin to the mechanical breakdown of chewing. Physically breaking up the chitin eases the burden on the stomach. Soaking the mushroom powder in lemon juice further mimics digestion, as lemon juice has a pH from 2 to 2.6, similar to the acidic environment of our stomachs.

**Effects:** Lemon Tek lessens nausea. It also causes a quicker onset and a noticeably more powerful and shorter trip. This occurs because finely grinding the mushrooms results in more surface area for easy digestion while the acidic lemon juice jump-starts the psilocybin-to-psilocin conversion.

**Mushroom Tea**

- Grind dried mushrooms into a fine powder.
- Set water to boil but be careful not to overheat the mushrooms or you will destroy the psilocybin. If you have a variable-temperature kettle, set it to around 158°F (70°C). If not, remove the water from the heat as soon as bubbles form at the bottom of the kettle.
- Steep the mushroom powder in the hot water for ten to twenty minutes. Add ginger if desired.

*CONTINUED*

- The powder can then be strained or left in the tea as you drink it, depending on your susceptibility to nausea. If you strain the mushrooms, you can wash them several times with more hot water.
- Effects will come on sooner, and the journey will be shorter.

## Mushroom Honey

Mushroom Honey is easy to make but requires advance planning—start the process about three weeks before your journey.

- Roughly chop dry mushrooms or lightly blend them.
- Mix them into honey, cover, and let the mixture sit for at least three weeks to allow the psilocybin to diffuse into the honey. Shake now and then.
- Once the Mushroom Honey is ready, add it to warm (not boiling-hot) tea, eat it raw, or spread it over toast. You can use the honey as is or run it through a cheesecloth to filter out the mushroom bits.

*Note:* Avoid powdering the mushrooms, as this makes straining difficult.

## Mushroom Chocolates

We can thank our Aztec and Mayan ancestors for this recipe. Mushrooms and cacao are both native to Mexico and South America and have accompanied each other in rituals for centuries.

Make Mushroom Chocolates by mixing dry mushroom powder into a chocolate base. The chocolate masks the dank mushroomy flavor and makes the mix more palatable.

- Melt chocolate separately and pour it into your chocolate molds first.
- Allow it to cool a bit before stirring in dry mushroom powder. This is very important—it ensures that the mushrooms don't overheat and preserves the active ingredients.
- Let the batch cool and harden.

*Note:* The better the chocolate you use, the better tasting your truffles will be. I recommend Guittard. It's a bit more expensive, but you deserve it.

If you don't want to go to the trouble, mix warm mushroom powder into a heaping tablespoon of Nutella and down it. It does the trick.

## Long Chewing

The simplest method of lessening nausea is to chew magic mushrooms for several minutes before swallowing, allowing the acids in your saliva to break down the chitin. This method is not delicious, but you'll likely feel less stomach upset than you would if you quickly gulped them down.

## PROGRESSION
## OF A TYPICAL JOURNEY

**Liftoff:** Forty-five to sixty minutes by chewing. Effects come on more quickly when mushrooms are brewed in tea or predigested in lemon juice.

**Peak:** Hours two and three. Mushrooms create a stronger body high than LSD or other psychedelics do, so expect to feel a lighter head, some disengagement from your body, and visual waviness. Mushrooms can induce laughter or deep philosophical or contemplative thinking. Go with it!

**Comedown:** Hours three and four. Effects will begin to fade, typically in waves.

**Landing:** Hours five and six. You'll be relaxed and your mind may feel full of thoughts, but they won't be insistent. You may be pleasantly tired.

## THE BIGGEST DANGER
## OF MAGIC MUSHROOMS

Most psilocybin-containing mushrooms are impossible to distinguish among the thousands of small brown fungi dotting damp forests and pastures around the world. But many of the look-alike species are toxic, and it takes a good deal of technical experience to differentiate magic mushrooms from other "trickster" species in the wild. If you're new to foraging, leave magic mushroom hunting to the experts. And be 110 percent confident in your identification skills before eating any.

## STORAGE AND CARE

Keep dry mushrooms in an airtight container in a cool, dark place. Light and heat can break down psilocybin, while moisture can cause mold. Avoid freezing, as the formation of ice crystals can damage the mushrooms. Desiccants such as silica gel packs can improve shelf life.

### HISTORY

Some historians suggest that North African and European cave paintings from nine thousand to seven thousand years ago pictured magic mushrooms.[3] Egyptian hieroglyphs pictured mushrooms with the domed cap and long, thin stem characteristic of psilocybin varieties. The Egyptian Book of the Dead calls these mushrooms "flesh of the gods." Thousands of miles and years later, the Aztecs were found to use a hallucinogenic substance in their rituals called teonanacatl, which has the same translation!

Artifacts and historical documents suggest that native peoples in South America and Mexico used magic mushrooms in religious ceremonies and in healing as early as three thousand years ago. They were first written about by sixteenth-century conquistadores, prior to the Spanish prohibiting their use. Although the conquistadores banned all entheogenic (God-revealing) plants in an attempt to force indigenous peoples to adopt Catholicism, native peoples continued using them ceremonially in ways that intertwined with Catholicism.

In the late 1930s, a young Harvard botanist named Richard Evans Schultes identified shamanistic mushroom use by native peoples in

Oaxaca, Mexico. Psilocybin was eventually isolated and then synthesized by Albert Hofmann in 1958.

Psilocybin was used in psychiatric and psychological research in the 1960s and was greeted with great promise as a treatment for depression until it was banned in 1970 in the US, and in the 1980s in Germany.

Research into psilocybin resumed fitfully in 1999; Roland Griffiths's landmark paper on psilocybin and "mystical-type experiences" was published in 2006.[4] Today, the synthesized psilocybin molecule (not the mushroom) is the preferred compound in psychedelic studies because it has a shorter duration of action and less notoriety than LSD.

## THE CIA BROUGHT MAGIC MUSHROOMS TO THE WEST

As a young man, R. Gordon Wasson described all mushrooms as "putrid" but that was more out of ignorance than experience. That changed when he fell crazy in love with his wife-to-be, Valentina, an MD and an expert mycologist who foraged fungi as a girl growing up in Russia.

Wasson's conversion occurred when Tina took him foraging in Eastern Europe. He became captivated by these creatures that are neither plant nor animal but form their own kingdom of life. Over the next thirty years Wasson became a successful executive—he was a VP for public relations at JPMorgan—and a full-blown amateur mycologist.

The couple read about teonanacatl, the "flesh of the gods" mushrooms revered by the Aztecs, in Richard Evan Schultes's work. In 1955 on a trip to Huautla de Jiménez, a small Mazateca village in Oaxaca, Mexico, Wasson met Maria Sabina, a skilled mushroom forager and *sabia* (wise woman). In a series of ceremonies, Maria Sabina gave him the secret, sacred mushrooms that her people had used for centuries in traditional healing ceremonies.

Back in the US, Wasson sent some of these mushrooms to Albert Hofmann, the chemist who first synthesized LSD. Hofmann isolated the active ingredients, psilocybin and psilocin, saw that they were chemical cousins to LSD, and tried them on himself. When Maria Sabina was later presented with a synthesized psilocybin pill, she took it and proclaimed that it contained the same spirit as her *niños santos.*

In 1957, Wasson wrote about his Mexico trip for *Life* magazine. That eight-page article, "Seeking the Magic Mushroom," introduced Americans to the fantastical fungi, which forever became known as magic. This brought a slew of other travelers to Huautla, where life was never the same, especially for Maria Sabina.

Wasson had agreed to keep her name and the location of her village secret, which he did in the *Life* piece, but the following year he revealed it in a book he self-published called *Russia, Mushrooms, and History.*

CONTINUED

The revelation proved disastrous for the Mazatec community, which, in the words of one modern historian, viewed the entire affair as "a story of extraction, cultural appropriation, bioprospecting, and colonization."[5] Mexican police accused Maria Sabina of selling drugs to foreigners; her fellow villagers, upset at the influx of drug-seeking tourists and the unwanted attention, burned down her house and murdered her son.

But here's the even crazier part: Wasson's journey was funded by the CIA.

In his *Life* article, Wasson wrote that his trip had been funded by the Geschickter Fund for Medical Research. Unbeknownst to him, Geschickter was a front for the CIA's MK-Ultra Program, the illegal human experimentation scheme established to identify drugs that could be used to coerce confessions during interrogations. The CIA hoped Wasson would return with "mind-softening" mushrooms. That section of the MK-Ultra project was abandoned shortly thereafter.

Years later, Wasson voiced regret at shining a spotlight on the Mazatec people and defiling their sacred ritual, and in every talk he gave he acknowledged his debt to Maria Sabina and his own wife, Tina.

## WHAT THE RESEARCH SAYS

### Psilocybin for Depression

*Note: All clinical trials use lab-derived psilocybin in studies, not magic mushrooms themselves.*

A 2022 Johns Hopkins study[6] reports promising antidepressant effects of psilocybin-assisted psychotherapy that last at least one year for some patients.[6]

"Compared to standard antidepressants, which must be taken for long stretches of time, psilocybin has the potential to enduringly relieve the symptoms of depression with one or two treatments," said Roland Griffiths.[7]

### Psilocybin for Anxiety

There have been thousands of anecdotal reports over the past sixty years of users eliminating or dramatically reducing anxiety with magic mushrooms. More recently, psilocybin-assisted therapy has successfully treated anxiety in people with end-stage cancer, as well as emotional trauma.

Studies from 2016 found that psilocybin can significantly and quickly reduce feelings of hopelessness, anxiety, and depression in people diagnosed with cancer.[8]

Another 2016 study compared the impact of microdosing magic mushrooms with that of megadosing on cancer patients with depression and anxiety.[9] Higher doses showed greater improvement in depression, anxiety, quality of life, and optimism.

This study failed to test the long-term impact of microdosing, but the benefits of microdosing are cumulative—they accrete over time. They would only become apparent after long-term use, not onetime use.

### Psilocybin for Alcohol Addiction

Most research on the use of psychedelics for treating addiction revolves around LSD (the focus of older research) or ayahuasca and ibogaine (the focus of newer research), but one 2022 study explored the impact of psilocybin on alcohol use disorder.[10] It involved two sessions of doses between 0.3 and 0.4 mg/kg of pure psilocybin (the equivalent of 4 to 6 grams of magic mushrooms).

Results showed dramatic reductions in alcohol consumption and cravings. Effects lasted through the follow-up period, thirty-two weeks later.

## Psilocybin Helps Longtime Smokers Quit

A small 2014 Johns Hopkins study showed that two to three moderate to high doses of psilocybin combined with cognitive behavioral therapy enabled 80 percent of subjects to quit smoking and stay smoke-free for at least six months.[11] For perspective, standard interventions with pharmaceutical medications have a quit rate of 35 percent and don't endure as long. A follow-up study at twelve months showed that 67 percent were still smoke-free, and all but two of the participants rated their psilocybin experience as one of the five most meaningful experiences in their lives.[12]

## Psilocybin for Spiritual or Mystical Experiences[13]

In 2019, Johns Hopkins launched an online survey with people who had used psilocybin, LSD, ayahuasca, or DMT. Most of the four-thousand-plus[*] participants reported vivid memories of their psychedelic encounters, which frequently involved communication with some entity they described as conscious, benevolent, intelligent, sacred, eternal, and all-knowing. Half of the people called it a "complete mystical experience." All had moderate to strong positive changes in life satisfaction, purpose, and meaning. Over two-thirds of those who identified as atheist before psilocybin no longer identified as atheist afterward.

The experiences of those who took psilocybin and LSD were most similar; the ayahuasca group had the highest rates of enduring positive consequences.

### The Six Most Popular Magic Mushrooms in North America[**] and Their Potency

| POTENCY | VARIETIES |
|---|---|
| Average potency (follow the dosing guides on page 68) | **Golden Teacher:** Gentle onset, more mental than physical. Easy to manage. **B+:** Good visuals and euphoria; may cause more nausea or lethargy. |
| Middle-of-the-road potency | **Penis Envy:** Fast onset, wavy visuals, minimal body load. Can be surprisingly strong. |
| Higher potency | These are about twice as powerful as those listed above, so if you're inexperienced, start by using half of the recommended doses. **Tidal Wave** (a hybrid of B+ and Penis Envy): Fast onset (thus the name); euphoria, strong visuals, and a steady current of mental clarity. **Liberty Caps:** More "head high" than "body high," with intense visual hallucinations. **Wavy Caps:** Powerful! Users describe high-dose effects similar to those of DMT, including mystical experiences. |

---

[*] N = 809. Psilocybin 1,184; LSD 1,251; ayahuasca 435; DMT 606.
[**] Courtesy of the good people at Third Wave.

## THE OVERLAPPING DISCOVERY OF PSILOCYBIN AND BETA BLOCKERS

The psilocybin and psilocin in magic mushrooms inspired Albert Hofmann to synthesize pindolol,[14] one of the earliest of the beta blockers, drugs that slow down the heart and are today a multibillion-dollar class of pharmaceuticals. So when we talk about plants or fungi of the gods, we're not just talking about compounds that treat mental or emotional illnesses. These compounds have revolutionized Western medicine.

## LEGALITY:
### THE LANDSCAPE IS CHANGING

Denver, Colorado, broke new ground in May 2019, becoming the first city to decriminalize psilocybin. A handful of cities have followed suit, and many more are expected to join the list in coming years. The state of Oregon decriminalized psilocybin in 2020, also legalizing supervised therapeutic use; there has since been retrenchment in certain localities. Colorado passed a similar measure in 2022.

Laws in the US and around the world are changing at such a pace that an exhaustive list would be outdated within the year. It's also difficult to stay ahead of where mushrooms are legal, where they're decriminalized, and where it's legal to possess small quantities for personal use. The Psychedelic Legalization and Decriminalization Tracker can be accessed at psychedelicalpha.com/data/psychedelic-laws.

## GROWING MUSHROOMS IS NOT ILLEGAL

While possessing and selling magic mushrooms is illegal in the US, growing them is not. A further complication: While the mushroom itself is illegal, the spores do not contain the drugs and are therefore not illegal.

# PAUL STAMETS: MUSHROOM MESSIAH

Paul Stamets has been a messiah for mushrooms (psilocybin and otherwise) since the 1978 publication of *Psilocybe Mushrooms and Their Allies*. He is one of the planet's foremost experts in psilocybin mushrooms: He has written seven books and initiated the "Liberation Mycology" movement that instructs people in growing mushrooms at home, in closets, basements, and cupboards. He also inspired the documentary *Fantastic Fungi*.

Stamets believes, and science backs him up, that networks of mycelium—the underground, rootlike structures of mushrooms—are sentient, intelligent, and have immune systems just as people do. Listen to any of his talks and you'll probably come away believing the same.

**As an entrepreneur:** Stamets founded Fungi Perfecti, makers of Host Defense Systems mushroom supplements and adaptogens.

**As a fashion icon:** Stamets rarely appears without his hat made from amadou, a spongy, inedible material that grows from *Fomes fomentarius* and similar polyspore fungi.

**As an ex-stutterer:** When he was a teenager, Paul took a heroic dose and climbed a tree. A surprise thunderstorm kept him trapped in the branches, tripping, terrified, and probably amazed. Holding on, he began chanting, "Stop stuttering now," between lightning strikes. After the storm, he climbed down, walked home, dried off, and went to bed. The next morning, he ran into a woman he had been attracted to. Instead of staring down at the ground, he looked her in the eyes and said, "Good morning," without stuttering. He broke his stuttering habit.

**As an innovator:** Stamets has explored technologies using mycelium to stop colony collapse in bees, is developing mushroom-based animal feed that upregulates immunity so that pigs and chickens can naturally defend themselves against pathogens and viruses without antibiotics, and has advanced the study of microdosing via the crowdsourced Microdose. me platform.

**As a (hopeful) futurist**: "It may well be that psilocybin is the medicine of our time for creating a paradigm shift necessary for us to have the intellectual capacity to offset climate change and create a future that is brighter and better than the calamity we are experiencing today. . . . We humans make too much noise. It's time to listen to nature. This is the greater truth."

**As an advocate:** Stamets is a vocal proponent of the "Two Eyes Seeing" philosophy, preserving and learning from the wisdom from ancient cultures while at the same time introducing Western cultivation technologies to indigenous people. "We don't deserve indigenous wisdom given our past behavior; I think we should strive to deserve it with our future behavior," he says.

# KETAMINE

## THE FLEXIBLE PSYCHEDELIC

-----------------------------------------------

A ketamine dissociative state is like putting your brain on airplane mode.

DR. LEONARDO VANDO, *psychiatrist and medical director of Mindbloom*

Ketamine is a mysterious molecule that isn't a classic psychedelic but exhibits some fascinating psychedelic properties. Originally synthesized in 1962, it has been used as a combat zone anesthetic, an antidepressant and painkiller, a suicide interrupter, a veterinary sedative, and recreationally, as a dreamstate inducer. Due to its approved medical applications, ketamine is listed as a Schedule 3 substance in the US.

Used clinically, ketamine is deemed safe and versatile—it mixes well with many medications and therapies. It was the first psychedelic to be legalized and approved for clinical use and is listed on the World Health Organization's list of essential medicines.

At low doses, ketamine induces a liminal state between awake and dreaming on the edge of anesthetization. People often feel loosely uncoupled from their bodies, which they describe in ways ranging from rapturous to numbing and unpleasant.

Higher doses can take people into a pseudo-anesthetized and psychedelic state, ranging from blissful to somewhat frightening. Commonly reported effects are looking at yourself from above, out-of-body experiences, and super-sensitized hearing in which low-level background noises like the air conditioner come to the fore.

**Also known as:** K, ket, vitamin K, super K, special K, Kit-Kat, kitty.

**Source:** Synthetic.

**Chemical name:** Ketamine.

**Drug classification:** Dissociative anesthetic; arylcyclohexylamine.

**Methods of administration:** Ketamine can be delivered via IV infusion, IM or subcutaneous (SC) injection, nasal spray, troches (aka lozenges), rapid dissolving tablet (RDT), pills, suppositories, transdermal patches, and nebulization, as well as intranasally as a powder (snorted). Its many methods of administration makes it a very flexible psychedelic.

*Note*: The advantage of the rapid dissolving tablet (RDT) versus the lozenge: It dissolves in two minutes whereas the bitter-tasting lozenge must be held in your mouth for twenty minutes. The downside? RDTs have a short shelf life and some of them, depending on the manufacturer, must be kept in the refrigerator or freezer away from sunlight.

**Duration:** Depends on route of administration.[1] *Intranasal*: 5–60 minutes. *Oral:* 1–2+ hours. *Sublingual*: 30–60 minutes to onset; lasts 30-60 minutes. *Intramuscular Injection*: 30 minutes to 3 hours. *Rectal Suppository*: ~2 hours. *IV Infusion*: Sessions typically last 45 minutes to 1 hour, but can be extended up to 5 hours.

**Open critical period:** ~2–4 days.

## RISKS AND ADVERSE EFFECTS

In five hundred studies performed over seventy years, there have been no reported fatalities from ketamine used properly on its own. In rare cases where ketamine has been associated with deaths, it is most often due to accidents, such as drowning or hypothermia, or mixing substances that are fatal when combined.[2] People have also died from taking high doses of ketamine and choking on vomit or suffocating from falling forward on pillows.

However, if you're using ketamine recreationally or outside of a clinical setting, be aware that it is more habit forming and psychologically addictive than other psychedelics like psilocybin or LSD. Let me be clear: If you have a propensity toward addiction or dependence with any drug or alcohol, if you feel an overpowering craving for ketamine, if your nose is inflamed from inhaling too much, or if you're having trouble focusing, ketamine may be a poor choice for you. Used frequently, you can build a tolerance to ketamine.

Repeated use is also associated with urinary tract problems such as scarring in the bladder, which can lead to loss of urine control and leaking. Long-term use might also cause anxiety, depression, suicidal thoughts, or memory loss. The eighteen hundred members on the Ketamine Addiction subreddit describe peeing blood, seizures, hallucinations, permanent kidney damage, and "K cramps" (severe abdominal pain), all caused by overuse.[3]

Although ketamine itself doesn't slow your heart rate or breathing, it's risky to combine it with depressants like alcohol, benzodiazepines, or GHB, a drug commonly used in chemsex. These mixtures can lead to blackouts, spinning, vomiting, erratic body temperature, and loss of consciousness.

## CONDITIONS ADDRESSED

Ketamine is indicated for depression (including major depressive disorder and treatment-resistant depression), post-traumatic stress disorder, substance addiction, persistent anxiety, intrusive thoughts, disordered eating, obsessive-compulsive disorder, and suicidal ideation. Dr. Gerard Sanacora, a professor of psychiatry at Yale and director of the university's Depression Research Program, says that as the research expands beyond depression, "the quality of the data definitely drops off."[4] This will likely change as more studies get underway.

## DOSING GUIDELINES

Dosing is particular to the individual and varies widely depending on method of administration, so talk with your provider about low, intermediate, and high doses.

Most standard IV doses are delivered in a clinic at 0.5 mg/kg (~1.1 mg/lb).

Many providers today are experimenting with more nuanced dosing regimens depending on client needs.

The guidelines that follow demonstrate this can be used nasally (usually with esketamine, which is sold as Spravato).

**Microdose: 5–15 mg, 1–2 times a day; frequency can increase to 4–6 times a day or as needed**

"I consider a microdose of ketamine like an antidepressant or anti-anxiety maintenance medication that people take every day," says Dr. Erica Zelfand, founder of the Right to Heal Clinics in Portland, Oregon. "And it works well."

**Low dose: 15–30 mg**

This dose is typically applied for social and recreational settings, where full mobility and body awareness are desired.

**Medium dose: 30–40+ mg, used in conjunction with talk therapy**

"This is not a full psychedelic dose," says Zelfand. "It drops a lot of the armor or shame around certain topics. People get a little looser and open up about things they haven't been able to broach. It's like anesthesia for emotional surgery."

**High dose: 70mg-100mg IM or 100mg+ when snorted**

The journey can resemble that of an IV infusion and is typically accompanied by a playlist and an eye mask.

"Patients don't talk and I encourage them to let it wash over them but then have a therapeutic talk session, either with me or a therapist, within 24–48 hours of the trip. The data shows that the window of neuroplasticity is widest then," says Zelfand. She notes that rectal administration is effective and long-lasting—sometimes as long as two hours—because absorption is slower. "It avoids needles, avoids the chance of nasal burn, and unlike the oral troche, has no nasty taste."

# "Ketamine is an incredibly safe drug unless you do something stupid while you're on it."

—DR. ALLISON WELLS, anesthesiologist and founder of Lone Star Infusion, a Houston-based ketamine clinic

## PROGRESSION OF A THERAPEUTIC IV JOURNEY

**Liftoff:** Effects begin at once, as ketamine enters the bloodstream. Peak effects are felt within five minutes.

**Peak:** At psychedelic doses, you may experience separation from the body or a feeling of weightlessness, floating above yourself. Visions, deep emotions, some visual effects, auditory distortions, and new insights are common. You may be tired or somewhat discombobulated immediately following treatment, but recovery is quick.

**Comedown:** Effects subside within ten minutes after the infusion ends, though it may take a couple of hours to reach baseline.

## PROGRESSION OF A LOW-DOSE RECREATIONAL JOURNEY

Used recreationally, ketamine is commonly snorted in small bumps or lines, or sprayed nasally at 15 mg to 60 mg. At low, measured doses, it rarely causes a hangover.

*Note:* "The difference between a goofy buzz and total body paralysis could be as little as one or two baggie-dips," one user said.[5] Moderation makes the difference!

**Onset:** Snorted ketamine hits in five to fifteen minutes and lasts for thirty to forty-five minutes. At modest doses, users report feeling light sedation, floatiness, or the sense of being surrounded in a pile of warm, fluffy blankets.

**Peak effects:** These can include sedation, pain relief, separation from your body (in a good way), euphoria. One user said, "The effects depend on your position: horizontal or vertical—I favor lying down and using it for sex where the distinction between my body and my partner's disappears."

Says another: "K can make both you and the world feel tilted—as if you're walking on an underwater treadmill pitched at a 45-degree incline. But you've never had so much fun walking up a hill."[6]

**Comedown:** Effects subside quickly; one user described the comedown as "feeling pleasurable lopsidedness."

## HISTORY

Ketamine was synthesized in 1962 by Calvin Lee Stevens, a Parke-Davis (now Pfizer) chemist who was searching for a less harmful derivative for the anesthesia phencyclidine (PCP).

Unlike other anesthetics used at the time, which kept people teetering on a thin line between life and death, ketamine was considered less risky—it doesn't lower breathing rate, heart rate, or blood pressure. It was considered so safe that it was called the buddy drug during the Vietnam War. Soldiers carried it into battle. If a fellow soldier was injured, an untrained "buddy" could inject them with ketamine and treat trauma immediately without other painkillers.

Ketamine was an outlier in the history of drugs because clinical and recreational uses were discovered almost in tandem. In 1972, a

## WHAT IS A K-HOLE?

If you take a dose of ketamine so large that you find it difficult to move around or see clearly, you're in a K-hole. It may be difficult to swallow, move, or talk; you may vomit. A K-hole lasts between thirty minutes and two hours. It can leave you scrambled and/or wobbly for a few additional hours.

Some people enjoy K-holes. One user said, "It can feel like an eternity, but never long enough."[7] Others find them scary or miserable. As Fatboy Slim put it: "Get the quantity right and Wow! It's incredible. Get it wrong, though, and you really do feel like you're dying.[8]

Many of ketamine's peak therapeutic effects are achieved by inducing a K-hole with a supervising clinician. This experience can be much more pleasant and beneficial when done intentionally and safely. If you're taking a high dose at home, make sure you are lying down, and ideally have a tripsitter present.

Mexican psychiatrist reported it as an accelerant for psychotherapy, but the War on Drugs made research impossible. Just a few years later, people realized that they could snort a tiny bit and have fun on the dance floor. As a white powder that was affordable, available, and short acting, ketamine became a popular club scene accessory.

Eventually, authorities cracked down on recreational use, and in 1999 the DEA made it a Schedule 3 substance, which of course drove its popularity to new heights. That same year *Time Out London* declared, "Ketamine is the new E!"

In 2000, Yale researchers reported ketamine's dramatic antidepressant effects, which at the time was game-changing. No new pharmaceutical for depression had been discovered in almost two decades. Since then, over five hundred clinical trials have shown its promise for a range of mental conditions.

## MECHANISM OF ACTION

Ketamine affects a different set of neurotransmitters than do classic psychedelics and SSRI antidepressants. Rather than interacting with serotonin, norepinephrine, and dopamine, ketamine binds and blocks NMDA receptors. This increases levels of glutamate and BDNF in the brain. Glutamate and BDNF are known as "Miracle-Gro" for neuronal growth. People who are depressed for long periods are said to lose neuronal connections; ketamine theoretically restores connections and leaves the body/mind more open to the impact of therapy, meditation, and emotional processing.

Ketamine feels distinctly different from other psychedelics. "Psilocybin or LSD are theorized to open windows to the external world in the thalamus. Everything you normally filter out is let in," says Dr. Leonardo Vando, a psychiatrist and medical director of Mind-bloom. But rather than leaving you overwhelmed by sensory inputs, "A ketamine dissociative state is like putting your brain on airplane mode. It maintains some functions, but it's largely disconnected from all the noise of the outside world and from your own mind." At the same time, you get a third-party perspective on yourself, which can create emotional and cognitive distance between you and your problems.

Dr. Allison Wells, owner of Lone Star Infusion, agrees that the dissociation helps people separate from their depressive or sad thinking patterns: "One of my patients said she can more easily watch her thoughts go by and be the observer, not the thinker. It allowed her to see that she is not her problems, or that they are not her. Over the long term, I think ketamine makes people less reactive. When you're soaked in adrenaline and cortisol, your synapses are really pared down and you may get stuck in fight-or-flight loops and rumination. With more pathways open you have more flexibility and you're not as stuck in negative thought loops."

Wells has treated over nine hundred patients with IV ketamine; her experience reflects the data gathered from research: 70 to 80 percent of patients receiving ketamine infusions experience a 50 percent reduction of symptoms of depression or anxiety by the second or third infusion. Many stay on maintenance doses indefinitely.

## TREATMENT OPTIONS

Because ketamine is such an adaptable drug, there are many ways of using it therapeutically. Some ketamine clinics are run by anesthesiologists like Wells who administer IV ketamine as a purely medical treatment, often without counseling. Other clinics offer ketamine-assisted psychotherapy (KAP), which involves counseling before and after sessions and over time. Studies show that this method has more durable effects.

### Clinical Intravenous Infusions

Intravenous (IV) infusions are often administered as a forty- to sixty-minute session at 0.5 mg/kilo. IV infusion allows a practitioner to increase or decrease the dose on demand. Ketamine can also be administered intranasally with similar results.

A session can occur with or without music. Most providers favor emotionally uplifting or neutral music that allows the mind to wander without pulling it in any one direction. Wearing an eye mask allows people to better focus on visuals and inner experience.

Compared with other psychedelic interventions, the treatment window following a journey is relatively short-lived—two to four days, versus two to three weeks as with LSD or psilocybin. Ketamine is not a one-and-done treatment. A common protocol is two infusions per week over three weeks, which are followed by weekly infusions for another three to six weeks. Over time, the spacing between doses is increased.

*Note:* Some people request magnesium with IV infusion to increase potency and reduce possible hangovers.[9]

To amplify benefits after IV treatment, Dr. Wells advises patients to:

- Meet with their own therapist for follow-up counseling.
- During and after treatment, limit screen time to two hours a day and delete social media.
- Meditate or do daily affirmations. In one *American Journal of Psychiatry* study,[10] even benign positive affirmations—video games featuring smiling faces and positive messages—were shown to prolong the antidepressant benefits of a ketamine session for one month.
- Do a body scan several times daily, walk in nature or do forest bathing (see "Integration: A Smooth Landing" in chapter 4)—anything that allows you to take in the present moment as fully as possible. The idea is to fire up and activate those new synapses and neurons. "You're rebuilding a healthy brain network; the more you exercise it the stronger your overall mental health," says Wells.

### At-Home Treatments

Ketamine delivered to your home is a lower-cost alternative to clinical infusions.* You must have a qualifying condition (depression or anxiety), but once approved you will receive a monthly supply of ketamine lozenges. Most companies offer Zoom visits with clinicians and regular assessments via questionnaires. There are several companies that supply ketamine by mail including Mindbloom, Joyous, Smith Family MD, and Wondermed; each has its own treatment protocol.

Joyous offers a low-dose treatment for depression or anxiety. Whereas a psychedelic oral dose is 400 mg or higher, a Joyous lozenge is 20 to 120 mg. This produces a state of "relaxed ease" rather than dissociation, which the company says "makes people more

---

* Even though patients say ketamine is a rare medicine that helps them with severe depression and pain, many doctors, including Dr. Wells, are skeptical of at-home treatment and advocate tighter regulation.

predisposed to a positive, even-keeled mood over time."

Mindbloom offers a high-dose solution, as high as the IV clinical formula, or higher due to the more limited bioavailability* of oral administration. The aim is to give patients a full psychedelic dose at home. "The content shifting that happens in a psychedelic experience is very valuable for healing and alleviating suffering," says Mindbloom's Leonardo Vando. Mindbloom operates more psychotherapeu-tically, meaning that intention, setting, and journaling are considered crucial to efficacy. An app helps people monitor effects and prompts them to journal. Patients also have the option to join weekly or daily integration circles.

There is no third-party data, but one study conducted by Mindbloom in tandem with university-affiliated researchers** showed 62 percent positive outcomes for depression and excellent safety.[11] Joyous has demonstrated positive outcomes of 42 percent.

## KETAMINE VERSUS SSRIS

Fifty percent of people who use SSRIs for depression find relief.[12] In many cases, it can take four to six weeks before results are felt, and they may be accompanied by side effects such as weight gain, loss of libido, or blunted emotions. When ketamine works, it works in a matter of hours, and the elevating effects persist for at least three days.[13] "This is potentially a life-saving medicine," says Dr. Gerard Sanacora, director of the Yale Depression Research Program. "It really was the first treatment that could fairly reliably produce antidepressant effects within hours, and definitely within days."[14] But he warns that ketamine is not a miracle treatment, and it is not for everyone. Relief is short-lived, and optimal dosing protocols are still being developed.

## ARE KETAMINE AND ALCOHOL UNEASY BEDFELLOWS?

Mixing ketamine and alcohol can often result in a night of puking, but a growing number of people report that ketamine, like other psychedelics, has inadvertently led them to pare down their drinking. "I used to go out and have sixteen drinks and do a bunch of cocaine and feel like shit the next day," one user told New York magazine. "With ketamine it was this total shift of: 'Oh, yeah, I can do this' [without other substances] . . . It still feels like stepping out of my life, but I also feel fine tomorrow." Randomized controlled trials support this finding.[15]

---

* Bioavailability is the amount of medicine that reaches the bloodstream.

** University affiliations include NYU Grossman School of Medicine and University of California–San Francisco, among others.

## K-SPRAYS

Ketamine nasal sprays enable you to modulate your dosage more precisely than you can by snorting powder, especially if you mix the spray yourself. K-sprays are more sanitary, convenient, and discreet. By keeping nasal passages moisturized, they also reduce the impact on the mucous membranes.

*Note:* Sharing nasal sprays carries the risk of also sharing bloodborne pathogens, so it's best to ensure you have your own *personal* snorting device; at the very least, swab the applicator with alcohol before sharing it with others. And if you're snorting powder, be sure to use a clean surface and an unused straw. Sharing straws or bump spoons can put you at risk of infections and other transmissible diseases. For extra measure, flush your nose with water after snorting powders.

### How to Make Nasal
### Ketamine Spray (K-Spray)

Making a homemade K-spray requires a scale, an oral syringe with no needle, and an empty spray bottle—glass is preferred to plastic. All of these can be bought online for less than $40.

As far as K-spray dosing goes . . . an easy method is to mix 1 g of ketamine into 8–10 ml of warm distilled water and shake it to dissolve. Assuming that each spray of your bottle delivers 10–15 mg, experiment with the following number of sprays for different effects: For a mini dose, try one to two sprays. A dancing dose is two to four sprays. A sex dose (in which you are mostly horizontal or thereabouts) is four to six sprays. A blow-out dose (in which you're definitely horizontal) is eight to ten sprays. Of course, the potency of your dose depends on the dilution and your tolerance, so be sure to test these portions on yourself in a comfortable and safe environment first.

## KITTY FLIPPING

Kitty flipping is using MDMA and ketamine together. MDMA encourages connection and love while ketamine in low doses reduces tension and increases mellowness. When you're kitty flipping, it's wise to:

- Have tried each substance individually so you understand what you're in for.
- Test your powders for purity.
- Begin with a light to moderate dose of MDMA (80 to 100 mg). Once you reach "peak" (after approximately two hours), take a small bump or spray of ketamine to see how you feel. Don't overuse K. Most people wait thirty to sixty minutes between bumps.

# DID KETAMINE KILL MATTHEW PERRY?

On December 15, 2023, the *New York Times* announced, "Matthew Perry Died of 'Acute Effects of Ketamine,' Autopsy Says." The world's media parroted the headline, but the story went on to say that the actor, who had a long history of drug abuse, was found face down in a hot tub and that coronary artery disease *plus* the effects of an opioid-antagonist, buprenorphine, which he took twice a day, contributed to his death. Yes, Perry was using IV ketamine to treat depression, but the amount found in his system was *ten times the amount* used to treat psychiatric disorders, which is very different from what is used in a clinical setting. US Federal officials have charged five people, two of them doctors, alleging they overprescribed and illegally provided the drugs to Perry.

Predictably, calls for tighter regulation of ketamine were raised. Some blamed his death on at-home use. But Matthew Perry's death was the result of combining too many drugs at dangerously high levels. As the Swiss physician Paracelsus wrote some five hundred years ago, "The dose makes the poison."

All drug use outside of clinical circumstances is controversial, but research indicates that when used as directed ketamine is by and large safe and it helps countless people contend with depression. Home use is also a practical way to help patients maintain treatment without having to continuously visit a clinic. "When prescribed appropriately, I would consider ketamine use no different than prescribing other psychiatric drugs like benzodiazepines or stimulants," says Dr. Jennifer Swainson, a psychiatrist at Misericordia Community Hospital in Edmonton, California, who has published research about ketamine's abuse potential, and has treated patients in her clinic with ketamine for nearly a decade.[16]

One celebrity's unfortunate death should not be a call to withhold life-saving medicines.

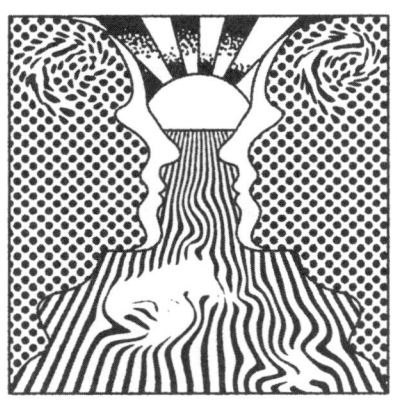

# DMT/5-MEO-DMT

## THE SPIRIT MOLECULE AND THE GOD MOLECULE

**D**MT is one of the most powerful, ubiquitous molecules on earth and also one of the most mysterious. The DMT molecule has been found in plants and in the blood, urine, and spinal fluid of mammals. It is produced in the human body and interacts with some system of receptors, but no scientist has been able to locate the DMT system or determine its function.

A close relative of DMT, 5-MeO-DMT is also found in plants, but it is most famously produced by one variety of toad that lives in the Sonoran Desert. *Bufo alvarius** produces a "venom" that, when extracted, dried, and smoked, creates an ego obliteration that has been compared to a near-death experience, bliss, or some combination thereof. If the impetus to chase down a toad to extract its venom, dry it, and then smoke it in order to touch God isn't a mystery, then what is?

Like skydiving or an orgasm, the experience of DMT or 5-MeO cannot be easily captured in words. Even though DMT and 5-MeO-DMT share a similar name and both produce brief, blasting trips, they are very different compounds. Molecularly, DMT more closely resembles psilocybin than it does 5-MeO. Their highs also differ. DMT is considered more visual, while 5-MeO is more somatic and mystical.

### DMT

**Also known as:** N, N-DMT; the Spirit Molecule.

**Source:** Many plant species, including *Mimosa tenuiflora*, *Diplopterys cabrerana*, and *Psychotria viridis*; synthetic.

**Chemical name:** N, N-dimethyltryptamine.

**Drug classification:** Serotonergic hallucinogen; tryptamine. Categorized as a classical psychedelic along with LSD, psilocybin, and mescaline.

**Methods of administration:** Smoked or vaporized; intravenously; orally with a monoamine oxidase inhibitor (MAOI), as in ayahuasca.

**Duration:** 5–30 minutes.

**Open critical period:** Estimated 1 week.** According to Gül Dölen, the length of the trip rather than the intensity determines the

---

\* The toad was originally classified as *Bufo alvarius* but has been renamed *Incilius alvarius*. Most people still refer to him as Bufo, and I will, too.

\*\* Dr. Dölen is often asked why she hasn't tested the critical period of DMT, which is unique in its intense effects and short duration. Her reason is largely technical: Her lab isn't set up to deliver vaporized DMT to mice, and oral DMT administration would require co-administration of an MAOI, as in ayahuasca. This combination regularly causes nausea and vomiting in humans, but mice cannot physically vomit. They would likely be miserably nauseous the whole time.

duration of the critical period. Inhaled DMT should behave like ketamine (short trip = short critical period), whereas in its ayahuasca form (DMT + MAOI), it should behave like psilocybin (longer trip = longer critical period).

## RISKS AND ADVERSE EFFECTS

There is one reported death from someone who used DMT in combination with 5-MeO-DMT.[1] The cause of death was recorded as "5-MeO intoxication." Another three people drowned while under the influence. Avoid precarious situations, and do not use either compound in or near water.

People with heart conditions should use caution with both DMT and 5-MeO as both briefly spike blood pressure and heart rate.

High-intensity psychedelics like DMT are not advised for people with a history of psychosis or schizophrenia.

Injecting DMT is not advised, since improper drug sourcing or injection methods can be catastrophic.

DMT should not be consumed with alcohol or stimulants.

## CONDITIONS ADDRESSED

Early trials are investigating the effectiveness of DMT therapy for depression.[2] Anecdotal reports, as well as success with other psychedelics, suggest DMT may be beneficial in treating anxiety, substance use disorders, traumatic brain disorders, and PTSD.

## DOSING GUIDELINES[3]

Depending on how it is manufactured or extracted, DMT comes as crystals, powder, or a soft clumpy material. It often has a yellow-orange or brownish color and a distinctive odor vaguely similar to shoe leather.

DMT and its relative 5-MeO-DMT are commonly vaporized in a glass freebase pipe. The vapor is inhaled deeply for about ten seconds. The taste resembles burning plastic. By the time of exhalation, the user is very far in outer (or inner) space. There are now DMT cartridges and vaporizers in the underground market that allow users to more precisely titrate their dose.

### Smoked

Threshold dose: 2–5 mg
Low dose: 10–20 mg
Average dose: 20–50 mg
High dose: 50–80+ mg
Shulgin dose: 100 mg

### Intravenous

Low dose: 0.05 mg/kg (0.02 mg/lb)
Average dose: 0.1–0.2 mg/kg (0.045–0.09 mg/lb)
High dose: 0.4 mg/kg (0.18 mg/lb)

## PROGRESSION OF A TYPICAL JOURNEY

**Liftoff:** Subjects in Rick Strassman's[*] experiments describe liftoff hitting with the force of a "nuclear cannon," "tidalwave," or "freight train."[4] The room may fractalize, breaking up into crystalline shards, your body following suit. You may lose awareness of your body as you become more of an energy speeding through a world of oversaturated lights, shapes, or patterns.

This rush can be overpowering and terrifying to the inexperienced, but then things open up—colors are electric, thoughts remain mostly

---

[*] Strassman, author of *DMT: The Spirit Molecule*, is also an adjunct associate professor of psychiatry at the University of New Mexico School of Medicine.

**DON'T TRY THIS ALONE!**

Due to DMT's instantaneous blast, it is dangerous to do it alone: You may be caught holding a smoldering pipe that could easily fall out of your hand. Use DMT and 5-MeO only in the presence of a carer who can maintain your physical safety.

coherent. One of the volunteers in Strassman's DMT studies described it as "a cosmic blowtorch, a tempest of color, bewildering, like I was thrown overboard into a storm and was spinning out of control, being tossed like a cork."[5] A color-blind user said he saw "all sorts of colors and shapes and weird objects."[6]

**The beings:** One of the more baffling aspects of DMT is the possibility of encountering "the beings"—also known as "machine elves" or "entities"—that communicate with users. They may appear as human, plant, machine, or insect and may predict the future or assist in working out a problem. People generally agree that they're "more real than real."

# DMT was known as "the businessman's trip" in the 1970s because it was over so quickly.

**Comedown:** The mind and the senses reconstitute gradually, which most people find extremely pleasurable. Visual intensity eases, and fully formed thoughts begin to return.

The landing is usually described as "clean." In another few minutes, you'll be either awestruck by the experience, effusive with gratitude and feelings of unbounded love, or absolutely certain that you'll never do it again. Many people described themselves as the observers of what happened while under the influence. They were surprisingly unaffected emotionally by the experience.

**Tolerance:** Humans do not build a tolerance to frequent DMT use.[7] Nor does DMT have cross-tolerance with other psychedelics. DMT is not considered addictive.

## HISTORY

Botanists first learned of DMT in the mid-1800s. It was chemically synthesized in the 1930s but largely forgotten about until the ethnobotanist Richard Evans Schultes identified it in the hallucinogenic snuffs of several South American tribes. These snuffs, called *yopo*, *epena*, or *jurema*, are mind-stingingly powerful. They are administered by one person blowing a large hit through a pipe into the nose of a recipient; the blast often knocks the recipient to the ground.

In the Cold War 1950s, Hungarian psychiatrist Stephen Szára attempted to buy LSD from Sandoz, but the company refused to ship it to an Iron Curtain country. Szára had read about the relative ease of synthesizing DMT, so he brewed a batch and tried it on himself, swallowing larger and larger doses to no effect. Only when he finally injected it directly into his bloodstream, bypassing the enzymes in his stomach, did he discover its extraordinary properties.

# "DMT is a tool, something to which consciousness hitches on for the ride. It might seem angelic but there's no guarantee it won't take us to the demonic."

—RICK STRASSMAN

In 1961, Nobel Prize winner Julius Axelrod identified DMT in the lung of a rabbit. It was later found in urine and mammalian spinal fluid, which qualified it as the first endogenous psychedelic.* The body does not produce random substances, so there could be a system of DMT receptors with which it interacts, but no one has located the system or determined what its function may be. Some suggest it is innately tied to dreaming, but there is no evidence to support that.

DMT has since been found in many plants (mostly from *Mimosa hostilis*, which grows in Central and South America) and animals—from coral-like underwater organisms to mammals that make DMT in concentrations similar to those of serotonin or dopamine. Because of its ubiquity, some experts, like Rick Strassman,

who studied it extensively in the 1990s and named it the Spirit Molecule, postulate that it is somehow intertwined with spiritual transmission and the very nature of life itself.

A Zen practitioner and student of Hebrew prophets, Strassman suggests there are two ways of thinking about spiritual transmission. The reigning biological model says that "the brain generates the impression of communicating with the divine, perhaps through the release of endogenous DMT." The other model, which Strassman favors, says that the DMT produced by our bodies "allows otherwise formless divine information to become perceptible." The more developed your intention, vocabulary, and other tools to mine the contents, the richer the experience.

In his book Strassman suggests that DMT may be somehow responsible for the way humans perceive reality. "The brain denies access to most drugs but it takes a fancy to DMT and allows it to cross the blood-brain barrier. It is not stretching the truth to suggest the brain 'hungers for it.' I know of no other psychedelic that the brain treats with such eagerness. Quick in, quick used, quick out. The brain burns it quickly . . . It is as if DMT is necessary for maintaining normal brain function."[8]

Imaging studies suggest that DMT shatters the brain's normal hierarchical organization and increases connectivity among regions, particularly those handling higher-level functions such as imagination. This ability to make thinking more flexible may be one reason why the early results of a DMT-assisted psychotherapy clinical trial for depression look promising. DMT offers one other advantage for clinical use: "DMT is short-acting, so it's a

---

* Endogenous means it is produced within the organism's body.

very flexible tool compared with psilocybin and LSD which can last for six to ten hours," says Dr. Chris Timmermann, research fellow at Imperial College London.[9]

## CHANGA: THE MILDER, MORE MANAGEABLE DMT

Changa is a blend of DMT and a smokable plant that is also a monoamine oxidase inhibitor (MAOI). Combining DMT with a smokable plant extends the length of the DMT experience by ten or fifteen minutes and also slows it down, so that the experience is more coherent than smoking DMT alone. Users say that changa has the same otherworldly aspects as DMT, but the onset is smoother, visuals are less fleeting, and users are more able to maintain awareness of external reality.

Typically, extracts from DMT-containing plants are combined with a blend of different dried, smokable MAOI-containing herbs, such as the ayahuasca vine and/or leaf from Syrian Rue, to create a blend that is 25 to 50 percent DMT. Changa is usually smoked from a pipe or small bong; an inhalation is held for five seconds or longer.

Changa was reportedly created by Julian Palmer, an Australian psychonaut, in 2003–04.[10] It's sometimes referred to as Aussiewaska.

**Risks and adverse effects:** Changa can exacerbate the negative effects of MDMA when the two are combined.

Like DMT, there is also an increased risk of serotonin syndrome when changa (or, more specifically, the MAOI component of it) is taken with many antidepressants, particularly selective serotonin reuptake inhibitors (SSRIs), serotonin-norepinephrine reuptake inhibitors (SNRIs), painkillers, stimulants, or 5-HTP.

## 5-MeO-DMT

*Important:* The following provides information on Bufo, but the toads and their ecosystems are endangered, so all users and potential users are urged to secure synthetic 5-MeO-DMT or attend retreats where synthetic 5-MeO is used rather than sourcing material from these vunerable amphibians.

**Also known as:** Five, Bufo, Frog, Toad, Toad Venom, Void, the God Molecule, Jaguar (synthetic).

**Source:** Various plant species; Colorado River/Sonoran Desert toad (*Incilius alvarius*, formerly *Bufo alvarius*); synthetic.

**Chemical name:** 5-methoxy-N, N-dimethyltryptamine.

**Drug classification:** Serotonergic hallucinogen; tryptamine, categorized alongside other psychedelics such as DMT, LSD, and mescaline.

**Methods of administration:** Smoked, intravenous, insufflated (snorted). There is an urban myth that "toad-licking," in which people purportedly licked the backs of toads to begin tripping, was a fad in the 1980s. This is absurd, since 5-MeO is orally inactive.

**Duration:** 10–30 minutes smoked, up to 45 minutes insufflated.

**Open critical period:** ~1 week, similar to ketamine based on duration.

### RISKS AND ADVERSE EFFECTS

**Reactivations:** One study reports that 70 percent of users have reactivations (once called flashbacks), but when used in structured group settings, they are largely perceived as positive or neutral rather than adverse.[11] Other estimates say that only 15 to 20 percent of people experience reactivation events.[12]

**Cardiac and psychiatric risks:** Bufo extract has a much more complex pharmacology than DMT. It contains a suite of other naturally occurring alkaloids and chemicals, including some that are known cardiotoxins. Many of these chemicals remain unstudied, and their individual risk profiles are unknown.

Do not use 5-MeO if you have a family history of psychosis, or if you have underlying heart conditions like arrhythmias or high blood pressure.

**Interaction with MAOIs and other drugs:** Unlike most other psychedelics including DMT, 5-MeO-DMT has monoamine reuptake inhibitor properties. This makes it dangerous to combine with other stimlants, even in separate but consecutive uses. Combining it with other drugs can have dramatic and unpredictable negative consequences, including cardiotoxic and neurotoxic effects, seizures, and serotonin syndrome.

Never combine Bufo with MAOIs. MAOIs are found naturally in plants like the ayahuasca vine and Syrian Rue (and other ayahuasca analogs that contain harmine or harmaline), as well as in a few prescription antidepressants. This combination can cause serious or deadly adverse reactions.

**Seizures:** On its own, 5-MeO (and particularly the Bufo extract) has occasionally and rarely caused seizures in some people. The risk is higher in users with epilepsy, who should strongly consider not using 5-MeO.

## CONDITIONS ADDRESSED

Like DMT, 5-MeO is in the early stages of being studied to treat depression, addictive behaviors, and trauma. One non-clinical 2019 study[13] with forty-two volunteers showed that a single inhalation produced sustained enhancement of satisfaction with life, along with easing of anxiety, depression, and PTSD. Another study from the same year yielded similar results with a large sample size of self-reported 5-MeO users in "a group setting with structured procedures."[14]

One 2020 survey assessed fifty-one US special operations forces veterans before and after a retreat in Mexico that administered 5-MeO-DMT followed by ibogaine treatments.[15] Respondents reported profound decreases in PTSD symptoms, suicidal ideation, depression, anxiety, and cognitive impairment, as well as increased psychological flexibility.

A small 2023 clinical trial[16] in Holland found that vaporized 5-MeO-DMT was "well tolerated and provided potent and ultrarapid antidepressant effects" in patients with treatment-resistant depression.

The British enterprise Beckley Psytech, in collaboration with King's College London, is researching the safety and tolerability of a synthetic intranasal 5-MeO-DMT for depression.

## DOSING GUIDELINES

5-MeO is ten to twenty times more powerful than DMT,[17] which makes it the most powerful naturally occurring psychedelic.

### Vaporized*

Threshold dose: 1–2 mg
Average dose: 6–12 mg
Heroic dose: 12–20+ mg

---

* Bufo extract, as opposed to pure 5-MeO, contains many other naturally occurring alkaloids and can be as much as 80 percent bufotenine (5-HO-DMT), a distinct psychedelic substance. Typical smoked doses of Bufo extract range from 60 to 100 mg.

## PROGRESSION
## OF A TYPICAL JOURNEY

Although Toad and DMT both begin with a blast—Michael Pollan called Toad "a Big Bang run in reverse"[18]—the visual field on 5-MeO often goes white. Users often report separating from their bodies as they travel beyond time and space. Some compare it to a near-death experience; others say it is "ecstatic," "blissful," "infinite love and peace," and "akin to seeing God," which is why 5-MeO is called the God Molecule.

The first mention of smoking Bufo appeared in an obscure 1983 underground pamphlet titled *The Psychedelic Toad of the Sonoran Desert*, written by Ken Nelson under the pseudonym Albert Most. Nelson was a reclusive psychedelic researcher, environmentalist, and veteran who lived in rural Texas. Due to its small print run, the pamphlet was only seen by a handful of people, but it has since been reprinted and is available for purchase. Following is his description of a Bufo journey.

An adequate dose for a normal adult of average size is a piece of dried venom about the size of a paper match head. Shave it into thin slices with a razor blade and put the pieces in a clean one-toke pipe fitted with a brass screen. Designate this pipe strictly for smoking toad venom, as the accumulation of residue in the bowl and condensation of vapors within the stem can yield an unintentional high with other smoking materials.

Apply a suitable flame and smoke the contents of the bowl in one complete inhalation. Try to hold the smoke in your lungs as long as possible as the effectiveness will depend largely on the full dose being absorbed in one breath.

Within thirty seconds, there will be an onset of almost overwhelming psychedelic effects. You will be completely absorbed in a complex chemical event characterized by an overload of thoughts and perception, brief collapse of the EGO, and loss of the space-time continuum.

Relax, breathe regularly, and flow with the experience. After two to three minutes, the initial intensity fades to a pleasant LSD-like sensation in which visual illusions, hallucinations, and perceptual distortions are common. You may sense a distortion in your perceived body image or notice the world shrinking or expanding. You may notice that colors seem brighter and more beautiful than usual. And, most likely, you will experience a euphoric mood interspersed with bursts of unmotivated laughter.

This ineffable episode is of extremely short duration [fifteen to twenty minutes]. The hallucinogenic effects dissipate rapidly and the entire psychedelic cycle is completed within fifteen minutes. There is no hangover or harmful effect. On the contrary, a pleasant psychedelic afterglow appears quite regularly and may last several hours to several days after smoking the venom.

A new edition of this pamphlet has been released with an introduction by documentarian and chemist Hamilton Morris. Proceeds go to the Michael J. Fox Foundation for Parkinson's Research, in honor of the author Ken Nelson, who died of Parkinson's.

## HISTORY

Indigenous peoples of South America have used snuffs from plants that contain 5-MeO-DMT for thousands of years, but today it's most famously sourced from a substance secreted in the glands of *Bufo alvarius*, the Sonoran Desert toad, which lives in the 120,000-square-mile desert spanning southeastern California, southern Arizona, and northern Mexico. For nine months of the year, these toads live underground protected from the scorching desert heat and sun, but the sound of the summer rain hitting the ground sends a signal to the toads to come out to feast and procreate.

Adult Bufos can weigh several pounds and grow seven inches long, making them the largest native toad in the US. Their olive-gray skin is slimy and leathery and interspersed with orange warts. They're ugly-cute but have become prized for the milky white venom contained in the parotid glands on their backs and limbs. The venom contains 5-MeO and another chemical, bufotenin, that renders the secretion psychoactive in humans. Until recently, it was thought that no harm is done to the toad when the venom is expressed, though that observation is now disputed (see below). Once collected, the venom is put on a glass plate and left to dry and crystallize.

One large adult toad yields half a gram to a gram of fresh venom, which when dried amounts to approximately 75 mg (ten to fifteen doses) of 5-MeO-DMT.[19]

Wider mention of 5-MeO occurred in 1992 when Wade Davis and Andrew Weil published a paper, "Identity of a New World Psychoactive Toad."[20] Davis and Weil had been curious why toads and frogs were considered sacred animals in Mayan civilization and why they so frequently appeared on pottery and artifacts. "The fact that this [chemical] exists in animals and is connected to the plant kingdom and to our own brains is very significant," said Weil.

### Legality and Sustainability

5-MeO was so obscure that the DEA didn't designate it as a Schedule 1 substance until 2011.

In states where Bufo is native, including California, New Mexico, and Arizona, it is illegal to collect, sell, trade, or possess the toad or its venom. Bufo is now listed as "threatened" in New Mexico and California, and transporting the toad itself into or out of these states is also illegal.

In the last thirty years, catching these fantastical warty creatures has become a popular but ecologically disastrous pursuit. The toad boom of recent years has led the already impoverished Comcaac or Seri people of Sonora, Mexico, to be threatened by drug cartels, which are profiting from the extraction of toad medicine and bringing crime to their homelands. Increased trafficking plus climate change and pesticide contamination further endanger the species.

Hamilton Morris argues that there is no sustainable way to continue the practice of toad hunting. He advocates using the synthetic form of Toad (5-MeO-DMT succinate), which provides the same high without hassling frogs or destroying their habitat. The venom is also an essential part of the toad's main defense system, so ridding them of it leaves them exposed to predators. Die-hard aficionados resist this, arguing that Bufo venom is a unique blend of medicinal compounds that create an "entourage effect" and deliver a more profound experience. But most scientists say there is nowhere near enough evidence to justify putting this species' survival at risk.

# DMT versus 5-MeO-DMT

Most psychonauts agree that people new to psychedelics should *not* start out with 5-MeO. Its intensity and potency should be respected.

|  | DMT | 5-MEO |
|---|---|---|
| Known as | Spirit Molecule | God Molecule |
| Where found | Plants; mammals; synthesized in labs | Plants; labs; Sonoran Desert toad; synthesized in labs |
| How made | Harvested from *Mimosa tenuiflora*; synthesized | Milked from toad; synthesized |
| Inhaled dose | 20–100 mg | 6–20 mg |
| Duration | 5–30 minutes | 10–30 minutes |
| Potency |  | About 10–20 times stronger than DMT |
| Effects | Very visual and interactive. People report visitations from other beings—machine elves, entities, and aliens among them. | "Content-free experiences" that are defined by detachment from self and/or environment, and sensations of unity with universe, connection with God, love, and other higher powers. |

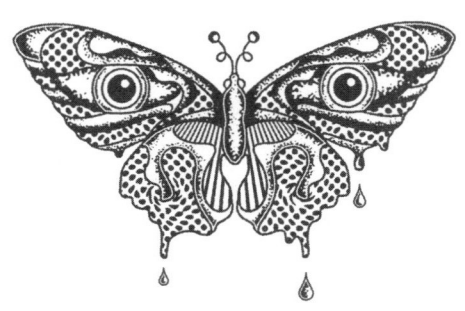

# AYAHUASCA

## THE MAGIC DRINK OF THE AMAZON

There is a magic intoxicant in the northwest Amazon which the Indians believe can free the soul from corporeal confinement and allow it to wander free and return to the body at will ... The Quechua term for this inebriating drink—ayahuasca—refers to this freeing of the spirit.[1]

ETHNOBIOLOGIST RICHARD EVANS SCHULTES,
*who spent fourteen years traveling the Amazon,*
*drinking medicine with many of the tribes he met*

Ayahuasca is a "tea" brewed with any number of psychoactive plants, usually containing DMT. Though recipes vary widely, nearly all of them include the bark of a gnarled woody vine, *Banisteriopsis caapi*. The most common preparation also includes the glossy leaves of the chacruna shrub, *Psychotria viridis*. The vine and leaves are boiled together for hours, sometimes days, into a thick frothing liquid. Other plants are often added into the mix.

Chacruna leaves contain DMT, but when orally ingested they cause no effects because substances in our stomachs called monoamine oxidases (MAOs) quickly break down DMT. This is why pharmacologists in the past insisted that DMT wasn't involved in ayahuasca's psychedelic visions. That changed when Richard Evans Schultes discovered that the *Banisteriopsis caapi* vine contains MAO inhibitors that prevent DMT from being broken down in the digestive tract. So it is the combination of chacruna and *Banisteriopsis caapi* that allows for the psychedelic effects of ayahuasca. *Aya* is the Quechua word meaning "vine of the soul" or "vine of the ancestors." About one hundred of the four hundred native tribes of the Amazon basin drink ayahuasca communally

**Also known as:** Aya, the Medicine, Grandmother. In Peru, Colombia, and Ecuador, it's known as *yagé*, *caapi*, or *kahpi*. In Brazil, it's called *hoasca*, *daime* ("give me" in Portuguese), or *vegetal*.

**Active ingredients:** DMT along with many possible naturally occurring alkaloids, depending on plant ingredients. These are most commonly harmala alkaloids, such as harmine, harmaline, and THH, which function as monoamine oxidase inhibitors (MAOIs).

**Source:** *Banisteriopsis caapi* (harmala alkaloids), along with one or more of the following: *Diplopterys cabrerana*, *Psychotria viridis*, *Mimosa tenuiflora*, other admixture plants.

**Chemical name:** N,N-dimethyltryptamine.

**Drug classification:** Both components are classified. DMT from chacruna leaves: Serotonergic hallucinogen; tryptamine.
Harmala alkaloids from the *caapi* vine: MAOI; beta carboline.

**Methods of administration:** Oral, served as a tea.

**Duration:** 6–8 hours.

**Open critical period:** Estimated 3 weeks.

## RISKS AND ADVERSE EFFECTS

Ayahuasca slightly increases heart rate but not as powerfully as DMT. Dennis McKenna suggests that ayahuasca, when combined with an SSRI, could cause serotonin syndrome.[2*] Some experts advise stopping SSRIs eight weeks prior to a journey. While SSRIs generally clear the bloodstream in eight weeks, Dr. Erica Zelfand has observed them to have enduring effects and advises proceeding with caution. "The MAOI in ayahuasca does not combine well with SSRIs and that drug-drug interaction can cause significant harm," she says. "*Never combine them.*"

Additionally, SSRI tapering should be medically supervised and can extend for months. It should not be attempted with the idea of attending a ceremony by a certain date. "The longer you've been on a psych med, the longer it takes to get off it, even if your depression has ended," says Zelfand. "Your brain has absolutely changed. SSRIs like Prozac or Lexapro work by keeping serotonin in the synapse longer. Your brain adapts to this by down-regulating serotonin receptors. If fewer receptors are being expressed and you taper too quickly this is a form of cruel and unusual chemical torture."

Another caveat: A medication taper is chemically, psychologically, and emotionally destabilizing, as is a psychedelic journey. Sandwiching the two can open a Pandora's box of trouble. "A lot of my patients who've combined the two later tell me it just wasn't worth it," says Zelfand.

Ayahuasca is not the only transformative experience on the planet. Psilocybin can be a gentler alternative, as can Holotropic Breathwork, which uses no substances and is said to produce powerful results especially when mixed with cannabis.

Finally, there have been reports of "false shamans" using toxic plants as additives to the brew (especially toé, a form of *Brugmansia suaveolens*) to supercharge the visuals for Westerners. Be sure to choose your medicine server carefully.

## CONDITIONS ADDRESSED

To those who prefer framing ancient wisdom through a modern research lens, two small studies focusing on members of the Brazilian União do Vegetal church (UDV) may be illuminating.

The UDV was formed in 1961 and has about twenty-seven thousand members in eleven countries. Many drink ayahuasca as a sacrament six to eight times a month in ceremonies they call sessions. A session lasts about four hours and involves silent meditation, chanting, music, and listening to teachings from church elders.

In 1993, a multidisciplinary team launched the Hoasca Project, a small study of fifteen men.[3] The results, published in 1996, showed

---

* Serotonin syndrome can present as a flu or an infection: fever, nausea, headache, malaise, tremor. But it's a syndrome, so it can also be extremely serious, landing people in a coma and at risk of death.

that ayahuasca caused no physical harm, nor did it cause any "neurological, cognitive or personality dysfunctions or patterns of dependency, abuse, overdose, or abstinence."

Users scored slightly higher on cognitive tests than nonusers. Many said that ayahuasca in conjunction with UDV membership positively impacted their lives: It enabled them to stop destructive behaviors such as alcoholism, violence, dishonesty, and infidelity, and live happier, more meaningful lives. Dennis McKenna, one of the study authors, noted that subjects had elevated serotonin uptake receptors, possibly indicating that long-term serotonergic modulation may reflect long-term changes in brain functions. Two of the harmalines in ayahuasca may also contribute to positive effects: Harmine is an MAO inhibitor that also stimulates nerve growth, and tetrahydroharmine (THH) elevates levels of serotonin transporters in the brain, which may contribute to feelings of well-being.

In 2012, researchers in Spain conducted a larger, more controlled study[4] with similar outcomes. These ayahuasca drinkers scored higher on perceptive and cognitive functioning tasks. Personality tests revealed them to be more flexible and less ego driven. They had fewer instances of negative thoughts and feelings and higher scores in "spiritual orientation," "purpose in life," and "psychosocial well-being." Results endured at least one year.

Subsequent studies have reported reductions in depression, anxiety, and addiction (alcohol, tobacco, and cocaine).[5] Researchers hypothesize that ayahuasca-assisted therapy may address conditions including PTSD, suicidality, eating disorders, borderline personality disorder, and Parkinson's disease.

## DOSING GUIDELINES

An average dose has been calculated at about 2 ml per kg[6] (about 1 ml/lb) but varies depending on the brew.

Precise dosing is difficult to determine, because ayahuasca is not one thing. Ethnobotanists have identified over a hundred different admixtures[7] that can be added to the brew, depending on the tribe and where they live. Most of these are flowering plants, but snake fangs, snake poison, and frogs can be included, all of which alter the experience. Effects vary according to method of preparation, setting, amount ingested, additional ingredients, purposes for which it is used, and ceremonial context, all of which are determined by the shaman serving it.

## PROGRESSION OF A TYPICAL JOURNEY

In indigenous as well as modern ceremonies, ayahuasca is administered by an ayahuasquero or curandero ("healer" in Spanish), who serves the tea to celebrants in small doses and drinks it him- or herself. People are typically positioned on mats. Blankets and small purge buckets accompany each position.

**Liftoff:** An ayahuasca ceremony begins with traditional prayers and *ícaros*, songs that healers use to summon the spirits. Liftoff occurs in thirty to sixty minutes and is often accompanied by *la purga*—purging. Shamans say that purging (vomiting or defecating) is essential to the process, eliminating toxic substances from the body. They also believe that many of the ills afflicting Westerners are the result of not expelling accumulated toxic impurities as regularly as they do. Indeed, small studies indicate that the alkaloids present in the brew can clear the body of parasites and other digestive maladies.[8]

**Peak:** The peak arrives at two to three hours. Plant medicines are said to have their own intelligence that communicates in an interior way, and what follows depends on what you bring into the ceremony. Visions commence, sometimes inducing fear, stress, and even terror. They are often followed by scenes of unsurpassed loveliness and spiritual illumination. Some people have transcendent experiences: conversations with plant or animal spirits, contact with a higher power, profound peace and ecstasy, an understanding of death and all that follows. Other people experience hours of physical discomfort. There is no universal ayahuasca experience.

**Comedown and landing:** As the peak slowly resolves, time is extended; visuals slow down and come in waves, eventually retreating as consciousness returns. Some people are drained and physically quiet. Many wake the next day softened or more vulnerable. Some people say their senses are more alive or sharpened.

## HISTORY

The origins of ayahuasca are impossible to determine because very few things fossilize and preserve the ecology of the rainforest. However, archaeological discoveries of snuff trays, snuff tubes, and snuff residue show that hallucinogenic plant use in the western Amazon dates back to 2000 BCE.[9]

Ayahuasca has been used by shamans to communicate with spirits during initiation and healing rituals and other community activities. Traditionally, the shaman would drink the medicine and then report what they saw to the community members who did not drink it.

Over the past several hundred years, ayahuasca has been integrated into folk medicine and spiritual practices, and today the community drinks the medicine.

Ayahuasca is used as a sacrament in three Brazilian syncretic churches, which combine indigenous and Christian traditions: the UDV (União do Vegetal is the largest), the Santo Daime (the oldest with a lively ceremony that includes music), and Barquinha (an Afro-Brazilian church). All three have now expanded internationally to Europe, North America, and Australia.

## SHAMAN VERSUS SCIENCE

Ayahuasca is increasingly used in neo-shamanic ceremonies throughout the Western world for spiritual exploration and healing, mental well-being, problem-solving, personal development, self-awareness, psychological exploration, and enhanced creativity. Dr. Rachel Harris, a Western-trained psychotherapist and author of *Swimming in the Sacred*, stresses that the healing that occurs with ayahuasca is not the same as a therapeutic intervention. It occurs on an energetic plane and remains a mystery to the Western mind. Accounts from scientists, ethnobiologists, anthropologists, as well as thousands of nonprofessionals, attest to its effects.

To write *Swimming in the Sacred*, Harris interviewed a dozen women shamans from various traditions who have been working underground in North America for twenty to forty years. I asked her how these women elders measure the success of energetic healing. "They know someone has healed when they see 'an existential shift in a way of being,'" she said. "They're looking for the inner spirit of a person to say 'Thank you for everything that is'

## ÍCAROS, THE SONGS OF HEALING

Healers learn ícaros during their long apprenticeships. They are said to be songs of the spirits that a curandero summons as allies to heal celebrants. They often have a rapid beat, which psychically seems to support moving through the flow of visions and minimizes the likelihood of getting stuck in frightening or seductive experiences. This is not the Western model of healing!

It's difficult to explain the power of ícaros, but the man in this video, who is married to a Shipibo woman from the Amazon, speaks about them eloquently.

See https://www.youtube.com/watch?v=r5P1RqUkzws. Watch his face when he sings. It speaks volumes about the power of transformative energy healing.

and to be joyful. That's really much different than what the medical studies are looking at. God knows we need the medical studies, but they're looking for reduced symptoms according to the DSM-5* and this is a completely different ontology."

Mark Plotkin, president of the Amazon Conservation Team and author of *Tales of a Shaman's Apprentice*, has spent much of the last four decades studying shamans and their healing plants from Mexico to Argentina. "These hallucinogens in the tropical forest permit medicine men and women to investigate, diagnose, treat, and sometimes cure ailments that have an emotional or spiritual basis, which is why they can sometimes alleviate a medical issue unresponsive to the therapies of Western physicians," he says. "In a sense, hallucinogens are vegetal or fungal scalpels which allow the shaman to find, analyze, treat, and sometimes cure emotional issues which our own physicians cannot."

### THE MYSTERY OF AYAHUASCA

The combined action of these plants has been understood by indigenous peoples for over three thousand years. But how did they select these two plants out of the forty thousand species surrounding them in the Amazon basin?

The standard answer from anthropologists was "trial and error." But as Dr. Andrew Weil said, "It's hard to imagine a shaman saying, 'Well, today's Monday, I think I'll try this plant and that plant.'" Instead, shamans say that ayahuasca gave them the knowledge. Weil and other ethnobiologists who have spent years in the Amazon lean toward that explanation, especially since there is no evidence to the contrary.

Even more interesting...although ayahuasca vines are botanically classified as *Banisteriopsis caapi*, curanderos classify them in more detail, based on their effects. Cielo ("sky" or "heaven")

---

* *Diagnostic and Statistical Manual of Mental Disorders*, the American Psychiatric Association's professional reference book on mental health.

ayahuasca brings one to celestial realms; negra ("black") ayahuasca is for darker shadow work.

## LEGAL STATUS

Since ayahuasca contains DMT, it is illegal to use in the US. However, in 2006 the US Supreme Court unanimously decided to allow the UDV church to use it ceremonially, since the US government failed to show that it had any detrimental effects. The Santo Daime church won a similar battle in Oregon.

Abroad, ayahuasca is legal in Peru, Colombia, Italy, the state of São Paulo in Brazil, Ecuador, and Bolivia.

It is decriminalized or controlled in Chile, Portugal, Spain, and Romania. It is unregulated and available in Costa Rica, Australia, and Argentina.

# THE GLOBAL AYAHUASCA PROJECT

The Global Ayahuasca Project (globalayahuascaproject.org) surveyed over ten thousand people from fifty countries, all of whom had drunk ayahuasca.

Many respondents reported increased mindfulness (acceptance, nonjudgmental and nonreactive processing, improved observation), along with greater cognitive flexibility and emotional regulation.

Broader reported benefits included increased confidence, optimism, independence, and positive mood, increased satisfaction with life, as well as more openness to therapeutic interventions and less anxiety and depression. They noted improved interpersonal relationships, sense of self, creativity, somatic perception, sense of connection, and a lowering of substance use.

Additional benefits cited: increased agreeableness, openness to experience, and extraversion, and reduced neuroticism and negative emotionality.

*Note:* If this all sounds too good to be true, remember that this was a self-reported survey, which means that those who answered were generally more prone to giving positive answers (those who had negative experiences tend to skip such surveys). Still, it is the largest survey of ayahuasca drinkers to date.

# INTERVIEW WITH AN AYAHUASQUERO

Being an ayahuasquero is demanding work. Leading a group ceremony while drinking the medicine and staying in tune with a dozen or more people all having their own intense experiences requires a keen amount of attention and focus. This is one of the many reasons it's important to ensure you are in the care of someone trustworthy and experienced.

Juan, who has guided a handful of ceremonies I've attended, is one such facilitator. A native of Argentina who today calls Costa Rica home, Juan first drank medicine twenty-four years ago and then trained for eight years with elders in Brazil and Peru. He is unusual in that he lives fully in the modern world, yet is deeply rooted in ancestral cosmologies. When I asked him how long someone should train to lead a ceremony, he shrugged and gave the answer that you should hope to hear from any medicine server: "I'm still learning."

### You don't call yourself a shaman?
No, I don't. Sometimes I use the word facilitator, and I'm comfortable saying I'm a medicine man or an ayahuasquero. I'm not crazy about calling myself a curandero. In Spanish, curandero means "healer." I have been a conduit for healing many times, but I don't specifically heal.

### How did you learn this?
It began in a different context, in the context of organized religion with the Santo Daime church. On my first trip to Brazil I met an ayahuasquero. I had a good connection with him and eventually I went to the Amazon assisting him, helping him out. I learned to do the cleanse and then to sing and then the tobacco, and I started going to the jungle every chance I had.

### How did you learn to make the brew?
He taught me the basics, but he told me that the final touch, you have to find that yourself. I started making it before even thinking of serving it.

### How long does it take to make a batch?
I usually go to the jungle for at least a week. Sometimes we go deep in the jungle, and we have to do everything: fetch the firewood, set up tarps, prepare a place where the pots are going to be. Once you get all that, then you harvest the plants. I go and I put my prayers there; I talk to the vine before we cut it. I do my offering with tobacco. That's how it was done in the past. I also clean all the moss and debris and the super-thin skin from the bark, which makes it a longer process. Then you beat it and cook it. It's time- and resource-intensive, but it's one of my favorite things about doing this work.

### There are a lot of reports about ayahuasca tourism and how it's depleting the species in the Peruvian Amazon basin around Iquitos. Do you always source your plants there?
I get them from Peru and I get them from another place that I don't want to call

CONTINUED

attention to in order to protect the plants. There are so many people whose spiritual lives depend on it and it's a bit underground, so I'd rather stay under the radar.

But in Peru, it is true that ayahuasca has become a commodity. You go to the jungle and tons of indigenous people and non-indigenous people are cooking it to sell and ship to different places. For them, it's just a way to make money. Unfortunately.

I still have tons of connections in the area outside of the tourist circuit, and they have a way of exploring one of the most intricate, intense, dangerous environments of the planet to find the vines.

**What led you to become a facilitator?**
At some point, certain spirits or beings sent a message. Then I talked to people I consider my elders, they were like, "Yeah, go ahead and start with small groups."

Looking back, I should have waited another two or three years. I had some major challenges because I needed some more preparation.

**When you led a ceremony that I joined in upstate New York, it was snowing outside, there were twenty-five people all having their own experiences, some quietly and some in loud distress. You drink the medicine and you're singing ícaros and you're playing your sharcap and other instruments, ensuring everyone feels safe and keeping the proceedings humming. With all that's going on outside and inside yourself, how do you maintain order and control?**

I compare it to surfing. The more in tune you are with the wave, the smoother the ride is going to be . . . but you never know.

You move your foot a little this way and you can go from having a blissful ride to getting caught and pummeled to the bottom by white water.

I can have sessions that are super fluid and easy and I feel like it's like a walk in the park, or I can have a session that I'm grinding and grinding and I can't feel it getting off the ground. And then you talk to the people and they say that was the most amazing, blissful ceremony. I'm like, "Okay, that's what I had to do for you to be blissful, cool."

**What purpose does singing the ícaros serve?**
It's a bit like sound healing, but we don't call it that. The ícaros are more specific. The different vibrations can touch different parts of our bodies—I'm talking about all our bodies, the emotional, physical, and energetic, spiritual bodies. They're all interconnected.

The ícaros are the connecting thread that binds these bodies with the medicine, the earth, and the cosmos. It's kind of like the ícaros have woven a grid, or they are making it evident, because that grid is there all the time.

They are waking up and activating all those threads that we think don't exist, if that makes sense.

**What language are the ícaros sung in?**
I sing in Spanish and Quechua. There are over sixty different tribes that traditionally

CONTINUED

work with ayahuasca, so ícaros are sung in over sixty languages.

### How many ceremonies have you conducted?
No idea. Several hundred, for sure.

### And they're never the same?
Even after all these years, I get blown away that I can drink from the same bottle on two different days and it can be so extremely different. We have all of these navigational skills, experiential knowledge, the dieta [food restrictions], the preparations, initiations, the connection with the elders, but drinking the medicine is diving into the unknown every time. Because of the innate wisdom and intelligence of the plant, you never know what you're going to get.

### After your ceremony, you lead a sharing circle, which is a nice touch but not traditional . . .
If jungle people had an issue after a ceremony, they can just walk to the medicine man's house and say, "Hey, let's talk about this." There is no separate integration because the ceremonies are a part of the community and part of the fabric of everyday life.

Integration is something we need in the hyper-individualized modern world. A lot of us are used to self-medicating, whether it is food, Netflix, porn, antidepressants, pot, cigarettes, in order to not feel things that are uncomfortable. And then you drink this medicine and it's like your sensory apparatus is getting upgraded or expanded or whatever, and it magnifies stuff you weren't paying attention to.

### I must be a super-messed-up modern person because I find that I'm still integrating for weeks or months after the ceremony.
There are a lot of tools . . . physical movement can be extremely important. For me surfing was my meditation. It could be knitting. Whatever puts you into that kind of one-pointed mind that's calming, doesn't cause stress, and has no agenda. Different types of therapy also can help you deal with trauma and heavy-duty processes.

### What do you advise people to ask when they're choosing a retreat or trying to decide who to drink medicine with?
You need to talk to people that you trust that have been to that place. You need to know who is serving the medicine. Do they prepare their own, and what do they put in it? You need to have referrals.

Now there are a lot of people in the Amazon catering to the Western mentality of wanting to do more more more. Jeremy Nardy [author of Plant Teachers] analyzed over a hundred samples of ayahuasca made by neo-shamans and found that they are making medicine with 50 percent more chacruna [the source of DMT] because that's what they think people are looking for. Or they'll do retreats where people drink ayahuasca four times in seven days. They're blown out of their shoes, and then two days later they're in an airport going back home. Some sort of confabulation is almost guaranteed unless you're an extremely grounded person and you have the discipline with your practices that will help you stay connected to your body.

# FINDING A TRUSTED AYAHUASQUERO

You wouldn't go to a doctor who doesn't have a license to practice medicine. So why would you undergo something as profound as an ayahuasca journey with someone you didn't trust? It's a buyer-beware market, so don't put yourself at unnecessary risk.

Michael Costuros, founder of Entrepreneurs Awakening, a psychedelic leadership coaching service, suggests looking for a guide who has had at least four years of apprenticeship under two or three teachers and who has at least as many years serving medicine to others. Ask the following questions:

- Have their teachers given them permission to lead ceremonies? The answer will let you know if the server is aligned with a lineage of healers.

- Does the guide visit the Amazon and continue their dieta under the supervision of master shamans?

- Where does their medicine come from and who makes it? (Ideally, the ayahuasquero makes it.)

- What does the guide get from serving the medicine? (Beware grandiosity.)

- If you are a woman and planning to go on a retreat, consult with other women who have been there before signing on to avoid awkward or dangerous situations.

# LSD

## THE MOST MALIGNED MOLECULE

-----------------------------------------------------------

I think that's the great value of LSD, that it loosens the constrictions of the ego,
allowing the parts of the brain that are normally repressed to be flooded with light
and things like the mystical sense can come to the top of consciousness.[1]

AMANDA FEILDING *at Albert Hofmann's one hundredth
birthday celebration in Basel, Switzerland*

Lysergic acid diethylamide is a synthetic tryptamine made from a substance found in ergot, a fungus that infects rye grain. It is also the most powerful, researched, and maligned psychedelic in the world's pharmacopeia.

**Also known as:** Acid, blotter, sunshine, Lucy, LSD-25.

**Source:** Synthetic, derived from ergot fungus.

**Chemical name:** d-lysergic acid diethylamide.

**Drug classification:** Serotonergic hallucinogen; tryptamine; lysergamide. Categorized as a classical psychedelic along with psilocybin, DMT, and mescaline.

**Methods of administration:** Oral ingestion* (generally sublingual).

**Duration:** 8–12 hours.

**Open critical period:** ~4 weeks.

### RISKS AND ADVERSE EFFECTS

The physical risks of classical hallucinogens, including LSD, are deemed minimal. However, these substances can trigger psychological difficulties including derealization, depersonalization, anxiety, dysphoria, and confusion. They can also exacerbate psychotic disorders or generate prolonged psychotic reactions if there are preexisting conditions.

No contemporary study has reported psychosis after taking LSD;[2] still, it's wise to steer clear of all psychedelics if you or your family members have a history of psychotic episodes.

SSRIs and MAOIs reduce the effects of LSD but are not considered dangerous when taken together with it. LSD should not be combined with tricyclic antidepressants or tramadol. LSD in combination with lithium can lead to seizures or severe dissociative episodes.

Since the 1950s, a series of sensationalized suicides have been blamed on LSD. The most notorious case occurred in 1953 when Dr. Frank Olson, a germ warfare scientist at the CIA, was unknowingly dosed with LSD by fellow CIA operatives in the clandestine MK-Ultra program. The US government claimed that Olson

---

* LSD should not have any taste. A metallic, bitter taste is a sign that you might have a different drug.

killed himself by jumping from a window in New York City's Hotel Statler. But two journalists, Michael Ignatieff and Seymour Hersh, who investigated the case separately, contend that the CIA murdered Olson because of the knowledge he had about US biological warfare during the Korean War.[3] The debate has never been resolved. But the night manager at the Statler who found Olson on the sidewalk remarked, "In all my years in the hotel business, I never encountered a case where someone got up in the middle of the night, ran across a dark room in his underwear, avoiding two beds, and dove through a closed window with the shade and curtains drawn."[4]

A 2021 review of the scientific literature[5] looked at sixty-four papers on psychedelics and suicides and found mixed, inconclusive results.[5] Some papers positively correlated non-clinical psychedelic use and suicides, some noted no influence, and many concluded that psychedelic use, especially in a clinical setting, decreased suicidality. The review concludes: "The results suggest that psychedelic therapy may be beneficial in reducing suicidality in certain diagnosed, clinical psychiatric populations and that classic psychedelic use may buffer against, and may be associated with reductions in, suicidality. However, within unsafe and unmonitored settings, psychedelic use can on rare occasions also lead to fatal consequences including suicide."

Tolerance to LSD builds extremely quickly. Sensitivity returns after a few days of abstinence. LSD is not addictive and has not been shown to create dependence.

## CONDITIONS ADDRESSED

Before Sandoz, the original manufacturer of LSD, halted production in 1965 in response to political pressures, LSD was recognized as a treatment for depression, addiction (primarily alcohol), and anxiety. Recent preclinical studies using another form of LSD verify its use for anxiety, but it has not been widely researched due to its past stigma that continues today.[6]

LSD is also used by people who suffer from cluster headaches and migraines. Cluster headaches are similar to migraines but more debilitating: They come and go several times a day, and each outbreak can last from fifteen minutes to two agonizing hours. Surveys gathered from Clusterbusters.org show that low-dose LSD (and to a lesser extent psilocybin[7]) as well as a non-psychoactive LSD derivative, 2-bromo-LSD,[8] offer significant relief for 67 percent of chronic sufferers and 75 percent of episodic sufferers. Interestingly, most patients report that LSD works better on its own without therapeutic intervention.

In 2001, Dr. Andrew Weil told CBS News that his cat allergy disappeared when he was tripping on LSD. "I was in a wonderful outdoor setting. I felt terrific and, in the midst of this, a cat came up to me and crawled into my lap. I did not have an allergic reaction to it and I never did since."[9] Weil theorizes that some allergies are learned. "That gave me the idea that [taking LSD] would be a great way to teach people to unlearn allergies. If the drugs were legal, I think I would recommend that some patients do it."

Dr. Weil's proposition has yet to be tested.

## DOSING GUIDELINES

LSD is the most potent psychedelic, so potent that it is measured in micrograms (mcg), which are one millionth of a gram. The most popular delivery format in the US is blotter acid, where a standard tab is (supposedly) typically dosed at 100 mcg. Other forms include liquid, gelcaps,

## IS YOUR LSD A LOWER STANDARD DOSE?

Emanuel Sferios, the founder of DanceSafe and the US importer of the QTest at-home quantitative testing kit, says that most of the blotter acid tested since 2023 averages about 50 mcg per tab, far less than the assumed 100 mcg dose. In his words, "Economics, even among psychedelic dealers and chemists, is a primary driver of behavior." Underdosing tabs seems to be a universal strategy for saving money and increasing profit, and it works because the market is completely unregulated.

or gelatin "windowpane," which generally contains up to 150 mcg per square.

### Microdose: 10–15 mcg
Sub-perceptual.

### Light dose: 15–75 mcg
Mild perceptual changes bordering on tripping.

One small 2023 study showed that low-dose LSD (26 mcg) elicited a "stronger positive mood" in people who were slightly depressed.[10] Twenty-six mcg is stronger than a microdose and may induce mild perceptual changes.

### Standard recreational dose: 75–150 mcg
This is a full dose, but not transcendent. You may get giggly, see visual patterning or pulsating (for instance, breathing walls), or have fast-paced and divergent thoughts. You're not "*tripping* tripping."

### High dose: 150–200 mcg
A high dose may bring on more stimulating visual effects and interesting thoughts. You can generally still be in communication with others.

### The Hofmann dose: 250 mcg
This was often the customary dose in the 1960s, in honor of Albert Hofmann's inaugural dose. It can start a transcendent, unity experience with intense visuals and ego dissolution.

### Heavy dose: 250–400 mcg
All of the above, plus you may disengage from your body, and standard logic may no longer apply.

### Heroic dose: 400+ mcg
Also considered an entheogenic dose. Body movement and walking may be challenging. This dose is for experienced users only.

### Massive dose: 500–800 mcg
Underground chemists working in the 1960s and 1970s experimented with doses of this scale. Some users recall rebirthing experiences, where you go down the birth canal

(and come out wet), death experiences where you feel your heart has stopped beating, or God realizations in which you think you're responsible for the sun rising (and at the end of the night, you're grateful you don't have that burden).

*Note: Only a QTest or lab testing can tell you the exact amount of LSD in a given tab. Dealers might approximate, but no one can know for sure unless they laid the blotter themselves.*

## PROGRESSION OF A TYPICAL HIGH-DOSE JOURNEY

LSD, like all psychedelics, is unpredictable in intensity and hugely context-dependent. Minor dose variations may also induce significantly different trips.

**Liftoff:** Effects become noticeable thirty minutes after ingestion.

**Visuals:** One to two hours. Colors are more intense, and the world begins to pulse rhythmically, as if it's breathing. This is brilliantly illustrated in an eye-bending video called "Forest Synesthesia" on the Qualia Research Initiative website. The creators of "Forest Synesthesia" describe it as "that moment when your senses start blending together and you realize that it wasn't a microdose." See qri.org/blog/replication-contest.

**Peak:** Two to five hours. Emotions may be strong, attention spans can be short, moods might swing, talking may be difficult, but words may not suffice in any case. Music can be enveloping. Euphoria is usually powerful.

**Post-peak:** The trip gradually declines in intensity until hour eight or so. If you have an appetite, some foods may taste amazing, especially sweet-and-juicy or sour-and-salty flavor

### PROPER STORAGE AND CARE

LSD is light- and heat-sensitive, so store it in a dark, cool place.

Also, chlorine dissipates LSD's potency, so use distilled water only when diluting for microdosing.

combinations. Emotions are highly sensitized. Be gentle with yourself and with others.

Comedown: Eight to twelve hours. A sense of emotional peace often follows, along with mental exhaustion or a slight headache. Melt into it if you can.

Afterglow tends to last most of the following day. The world may look flossed and polished.

### HISTORY

When discovered in the 1940s, LSD was thought to be a "psychomimetic" chemical that mimicked insanity. Sandoz (now Novartis) distributed it for free under the name Delysid to psychotherapists, psychiatrists, and researchers to test on themselves and patients.

Though the psychomimetic theory was ultimately abandoned, LSD sparked a sensation in scientific circles. LSD was discovered at virtually the same time serotonin was identified, and the structural similarities between LSD and serotonin, noted by the biochemist Dr. Dilworth Wayne Woolley,* led to a revolution in neuroscience that continues today.[11]

---

* Dr. Woolley suffered from severe diabetes and was completely blind from age twenty-five until his death. Despite his disability, he "saw" serotonin in the molecular structure of LSD. He was known by friends and collaborators to form detailed visual impressions in his mind's eye.

From the mid-1940s through the 1970s, over a thousand papers were written about LSD's therapeutic applications. In early experiments, the importance of set and setting on the user's experience was unknown, which caused confusion and wildly different experimental outcomes. In his first LSD experience, Dr. Stanislav Grof was given a high dose of LSD and then blasted with strobe lights to test his brainwave patterns. That sounds like the making of a nightmare trip, but Grof was apparently undeterred as he went on to administer over four thousand LSD treatments and write extensively about its therapeutic uses.

Early experiments produced two forms of LSD-assisted psychotherapy. Psycholytic therapy was mainly practiced in Europe. Patients were given low to moderate doses (25 to 200 mcg) accompanied by talk therapy sessions. North Americans used psychedelic therapy, which blasted people with one or two high doses in the hope of triggering a mystical experience that would catalyze changes in the patient's value system and self-image.

In addition to its therapeutic value, many deem LSD to be the grande dame of psychedelics and say it has had lasting impact on their lives and on culture at large.

Steve Jobs dropped acid ten to fifteen times between 1972 and 1974. He deemed those trips "one of the two or three more important things" he had done in his very accomplished life. (He added that Bill Gates would "be a broader guy if he had dropped acid once.")[12]

Kary Mullis was the Nobel Prize–winning scientist who invented the polymerase chain reaction (PCR) technique, an invaluable method for DNA research. When the BBC asked if his achievement would have been possible

# "Cars are real. Cliffs are real. Cops are real. You cannot fly. It's never a good time to die. And don't forget: You will eventually come down."

—Trip wisdom from back in the day

without LSD, he said, "I doubt it. I seriously doubt it."[13]

Francis Crick, another Nobel Prize winner, told people (but never publicly disclosed) that he discovered the double-helix structure of DNA in 1953 while taking small doses of LSD. Crick and his group of Cambridge academics reportedly used low doses as "thinking tools" to free them from preconceptions and let their minds wander to new ideas. When a reporter called to confirm the story, Crick sniped, "Print a word of it and I'll sue."[14]

In his book *Blotter: The Untold Story of an Acid Medium*, cultural historian Erik Davis called LSD "the twentieth century's most powerful technology of the sacred." Indeed, LSD catalyzed postwar 1960s culture more than any one movement in art, literature, and music.[15] Woodstock, Day-Glo art, flotation tanks, the Beatles (*Revolver*, the first psychedelic album, was written while the band was tripping—but don't forget *Sgt. Pepper's Lonely Hearts Club Band*, *Magical Mystery Tour*, and *Yellow Submarine*, the album and the movie), Charles Mingus, the Yardbirds, *Hair*, the Doors, Bob Dylan, Sigmar Polke, Andreas Gursky, the Dead, the Who, Peter Max, Burning Man, Stanislav Grof, Ram Dass, Hunter S. Thompson, Allen Ginsberg, Ken Kesey, *One Flew Over the Cuckoo's Nest*, *Easy Rider*, *Fear and Loathing in Las Vegas*, *Be Here Now*, *The Electric Kool-Aid Acid Test*, Pablo Amaringo, Led Zeppelin, Giorgio de Chirico, Robert Crumb, Roger Dean, Brian Wilson, Pink Floyd, Henri Michaux, Ray Charles, Eric Clapton, John Coltrane, Jimi Hendrix, Gilbert Baker (creator of the LGBTQ flag, who received his rainbow vision while high on acid and glitter at a San Francisco club), and the entire insane $1-trillion-plus War on Drugs, which fueled the underground—is any more proof of its incendiary influence required?

## MECHANISM OF ACTION

LSD has a high affinity for binding at the serotonin 1A and 2A receptors in the frontal cortex but also to other receptors found throughout the brain. Its pharmacological action involves serotonin, dopamine, glutamate, and noradrenaline neural pathways. Its close structural resemblance to serotonin enables it to attach to the receptor longer than the serotonin produced by our bodies, which explains the ten-to-twelve-hour length of an LSD trip.

## LSD: EFFECTS WORTH NOTING

- True hallucinations, where a person sees things that are not there, are rare. More accurately, LSD produces visual effects that range from fractals, patterning, or

## HOW IS BLOTTER MADE?

"Dipping whole sheets of [absorbent] paper into a bath of LSD distributes the material quickly and offers good control over dosage. The simplest method involves laying perforated sheets flat into a rimmed cookie sheet filled with LSD in solution, then drying them in air or on plastic. The process can be messy, which makes tripping balls a real workplace hazard. A more hermetic method involves sealing the sheets in a thick polyethylene bag with the solvent which is allowed to evaporate before the bag is opened. Up to 400 sheets can be dosed at once using these 'turkey bags.'"[16]

pulsing to full-blown changes in how a space, object, or living being appears. Sound can also be strangely amplified.

- While LSD is mythically all about the visuals, big changes also occur in perception of self and environment. Familiar spaces might feel new or alien, and it can be difficult to follow conversations or read other people's emotions.
- Some find the experience of LSD to be sociable and silly; others prefer to be alone or in less stimulating environments.
- LSD is described as "colder" and "bitchier" than psilocybin's "warmer," "kinder" profile. Strong emotional sensitivity can arise, which can be cathartic, transformative, or uncomfortable. At the

same time, the LSD experience is said to be less interpersonally involving, which may make it better for viewing art or taking in culture.

## CANDY FLIPPING

LSD can be mixed with other psychoactives for a kaleidoscopic array of sensations. Candy flipping involves taking a moderate dose of LSD (about 80 mcg if 100 mcg is your standard dose) and once it's doing its thing, following it three or four hours later with a moderate dose of MDMA (60 to 80 mg if 120 mg is your standard dose). LSD instigates visual and other sensations; MDMA adds a jolt of positivity to the proceedings.

Approach candy flipping with respect. Be sure to try each drug separately before you flip so you have a sense of what you're in for. It's also wise to use lower doses of each, not your standard doses.

---

## BEFORE TIMOTHY LEARY, CARY GRANT WAS THE PIED PIPER FOR LSD

Between 1958 and 1961, the Hollywood screen legend Cary Grant had over a hundred weekly guided LSD therapy sessions with Dr. Mortimer Hartman at the Psychiatric Institute of Beverly Hills.[17] Grant was one of Hollywood's most suave leading men, but he suffered from withering insecurity and depression throughout his life. LSD, he said, saved him. It enabled him to relax his conscious controls and reach his subconscious. Grant was extremely private—he rarely spoke to the press—but after taking acid, he did an about-face and gave interviews to several magazines, *Good Housekeeping* among them. Overnight, five million readers were introduced to the phrase *psychedelic therapy.*

Fellow celebrity Esther Williams read Grant's account and signed on for LSD therapy, calling it "the most amazing journey of my life."

Grant's LSD sessions occurred when he was filming *North by Northwest,* the period of his career that coincided with his box-office ascendance. Coincidence? Who knows, but upon his death in 1986, Grant gifted $20,000 to his psychiatrist as thanks.

# IS THERE A FUTURE FOR LSD?
## AN INTERVIEW WITH THE LEGENDARY WILLIAM LEONARD PICKARD

William Leonard Pickard is a former drug policy fellow at Harvard University's Kennedy School of Government and currently a research affiliate at Harvard Law School's Petrie-Flom Center for Health Law Policy, Biotechnology, and Bioethics. In 1996, his research into morphine analogs led him to presciently warn that fentanyl, then a rarely used anesthetic, would make a "perfect storm for unscrupulous manufacture," and would become the next major drug of abuse.

In 2000, Pickard was arrested and accused of manufacturing four hundred million doses of LSD in a reconditioned missile factory in Kansas.* He was given two life sentences without parole and served twenty years in maximum-security federal prison before being released in 2020. His novel, *The Rose of Paracelsus: On Secrets & Sacraments*, written in pencil while he was imprisoned, is published by Synergetic Press.

Pickard is currently the scientific adviser to a venture capital firm that is focused on next-generation psychedelics, neuroimaging, neuromodulation, virtual reality, and body wearables. The following interview is culled from a series of conversations we had by Zoom from his home in Santa Fe, New Mexico.

**Leonard, I'm happy to see you're in a beautiful place, Santa Fe. How are you occupying your time?**

*I'm a scientific adviser to the JLS Fund in New York City and I write blog pieces on biotech CEOs for Harvard Law. In my off time I take long baths (unhandcuffed), listen to classical music, and read. I just found a lovely old copy of Thomas Macaulay's* History of England. *I prefer early British literature. When I was in prison I had a steady supply from friends, so I had a book in my hand twenty-four hours a day. When I looked up it was tattooed thugs stabbing each other. When I looked down, I was in nineteenth-century England, with carriages and horses. I spent a lot of time in nineteenth-century England.*

**When was your last LSD experience?**

*I haven't used anything in forty years. Coffee is my last drug. I quit it occasionally then go back to it. But no psychedelics, no alcohol.*

**Why is that?**

*I made the choice long before I was in prison, because dealing with the energy that was required at the time was quite serious. It was a dedication. It wasn't a frivolous thing. I didn't want to be respon-sible for any state of impurity, or for*

CONTINUED

---

* Pickard maintains his innocence. His legal case is complex and he speaks very intentionally, a habit no doubt developed over a lifetime of discretion.

*doing anything in a cavalier manner. I wanted to go at it with absolute clarity.*

## What was the motivation of underground chemists working in the late 1960s and '70s? The risks were so enormous.

*If I had to address why people do that sort of thing . . . They thought these substances had effects that were very important for many people to experience: insight, an appreciation of the environment, com- passion for others, tolerance, a vision of what we could be as a species if we were more loving [or] creative or if we could use our greatest faculties to do good in the world. They didn't like war or the war machine. They didn't like outright greed and materialism or hatred.*

*They thought that these substances were a key to a new type of person, a new type of mind.*

*With that as a central thesis, there was nothing to do but synthesize large quan- tities [of LSD] and share them . . . and so people did. They saw them as a sacrament.*

## Do you still believe that psychedelics are a way forward for mankind?

*Psychedelics, I think, are a stepping stone. We're realizing that our perceptions and values can be neurochemically altered, and this opens the door to what we will do with this knowledge. We can change the direc- tion of our species. The question was then as it is now, "Who do we want to be, what kind of human do we want to be next?"*

## And who gets to control those changes?

*Right. Is it the government or is it a few pharmaceutical firms or will things run wild and free in the streets as they have with previous compounds? I suspect we'll see quite some changes with a drug that enhances intelligence or higher cognitive faculties. These are the drugs of the post- psychedelic era, things that improve skills, productivity, focus. My study of the literature suggests such a pill is coming.*

## Is LSD an easy drug to synthesize?

*It's certainly more complicated than methamphetamine. It can be synthesized by any organic chemistry major if they have a cookbook recipe, but the primary limiting factor is that the precursor chemicals [ergotamine and other ergot alkaloids] are very difficult to obtain. There are about twenty thousand kilograms of the precursors made worldwide each year and distribution is very tightly controlled internationally, so secreting a few kilos away from that system is an art in itself. A second factor is that it's quite another thing to go from an organic chemistry student making a black liquid or a gum that is 60 percent LSD to making kilograms of pure white crystal. That requires special techniques and processes, training, and dedication.*

## Do you miss being a chemist?

*To observe one property changing into an entirely different property is a beautiful thing. We do understand a small fragment*

*CONTINUED*

of nature and reality. That little we can understand has no less beauty than that which remains unknown.

In terms of LSD synthesis, the climactic moment occurs when you have a reaction going in a twenty-liter spherical glass container, and within that is what would become, say, ten million doses. It's swirling about under argon or some inert gas, bathed in red light because white light damages the molecule, and one is wearing protective garments such as a moon suit to limit exposure, and all this is going on in some secret environment, and suddenly, in a period of twenty minutes the entire ten million doses become psychoactive. It goes from just a swirling mixture to something that affects millions of people.

**You said you saw this chemical transformation as a sacrament?**
There are only a handful of people that do those kinds of quantities but among those who do, it's not uncommon to offer prayers that this will be a blessed event in people's lives. You can't let it go out any other way—that would be criminal.

That's how the underground functioned, so it's interesting these days to see the big corporations about to synthesize psilocybin or ibogaine, perhaps in Guangzhou, China, where a technician making this substance goes home at five o'clock and has no idea what it does. No prayers or reverence, it's just a job.

It's going to be very interesting to watch all that happen.

**Sounds fucking terrifying to me.**
I much prefer the former way.

There are people who say that the spirit of the molecule will not yield or come into being without certain reverence toward what is being done; that strange things happen, like people become addicted or people die or get arrested, or the synthesis won't work no matter if it's technically followed precisely.

Of course these are just theories . . . rumors and gossip from the underground.

## "In the space of a few minutes it goes from just a swirling mixture to something that can affect millions of people."

**And the downsides of psychedelics?**
A strong drug experience of any kind can also make one much less effective, incapacitated. If these things are used, they should be used infrequently, in moderate doses, and with intent. Not to just dance in the street, but with something that is arguably sacred, to use the energy

CONTINUED

for healing, to make humankind better somehow.

### Given its cultural and historical baggage, is there a future for LSD?

Indeed, there is. MindMed, which launched in 2018 and is today valued at $300 million, just got FDA permission for MM120, which is LSD for treatment of anxiety. There's always been a place for it. [For] quite a few elders in our society, their favorite drug remains LSD. Young people, too.

### MM120 sounds like LSD without the baggage of LSD, without even the baggage of the name of LSD. How is it different from good old LSD?

It's just a different crystal formation [known as] LSD tartrate. The tartrate makes it a soluble white powder. The beauty is that different salts can be patented. It's what the psychedelic biotech start-up Compass Pathways did with psilocybin, they came up with a salt form of it. It doesn't prevent anyone else from making their own salt and having their own patent.

### Your role at JLS Fund gives you a bird's-eye view into the future. How is artificial intelligence influencing modern drug development?

Things are accelerating as in no point in history. It is enabling Big Pharma to get past the one-molecule-at-a-time drug development that currently takes ten years and costs billions. The new methods shorten ten years of development to eighteen months.

We will see tens of thousands of analogs. Ninety-nine percent of them will be forgotten, but we'll have some new discoveries that will be quite amazing, some benevolent and some very dangerous. The future is both frightening and glorious.

### A lot of companies are trying to engineer the trip out of psychedelic analogs. What's your gut, can healing occur without the trip?

Being an old hippie, my intuitive feeling is that the long night of the soul, ego dissolution, the ineffable, are linked to the healing aspects.

But if we can have non-psychedelic medicine that works as effectively or more than existing remedies, my position is whatever works is very much welcome, psychedelic or not. Depression, Parkinson's, addiction . . . these diseases are not presently treatable with great success.

The medical model redeems this class of compounds in the eyes of the public. But before he died, Roland Griffiths of Johns Hopkins said he hoped these things didn't end up entirely in the hands of the medical community. He respected the non-medical applications for those who may want to nibble a mushroom, wander the forest, or just explore or savor the aesthetics of life.

### Hippies were blamed for a lot of things that happened, but I think they gave the world incredible insights.

We had this advanced neurochemical first deployed widely in a youthful generation.

*CONTINUED*

*There were no elders to talk to; we just spoke with each other. And these substances produced profound changes in music, politics, writing, the sciences. Back in the day, you integrated with friends. No one was presenting as "I'm depressed." Psychedelics weren't given to people who were unstable, since you knew you were going to have a very arduous night bringing them back to reality.*

*Today, there's so much happening that's truly extraordinary. Worldwide communications, billions of people online, the advent of artificial intelligence and genomics. There has never been a more exciting time in history. It is a privilege to witness.*

# PEYOTE/MESCALINE/ HUACHUMA

## OUR CACTUS ALLIES

------------------------------------

**M**escaline is the naturally occurring ingredient in peyote and San Pedro cactuses, two of the oldest plant psychedelics used by humans. Mescaline also served as the starting point from which Alexander Shulgin synthesized many of the other novel phenethylamines that he documented in his 1991 book, *PiHKAL*. Whether it occurs naturally in cactuses or it is synthesized in a lab, mescaline is known as one of the gentler, more insightful psychedelics, with greater emphasis on bodily or tactile sensations rather than the busy headspace or frenetic visuals associated with tryptamines such as psilocybin or DMT.

Synthetic mescaline is typically produced in small batches and incurs a high production cost, which makes it highly sought after by aficionados. Peyote is similarly difficult to come across due to its long twenty-year maturation, ecologically endangered growing areas, and protected status as a sacrament in the Native American Church (NAC).

### Peyote: "The Plant That Fills the Eyes with Marvels"*

Peyote is a small, spineless grayish-green cactus native to the Rio Grande Valley region of southeastern New Mexico, Texas, and north-central Mexico. Peyote grows glacially slowly in chalky, clay soils and often together in groups of around fifty plants. Maturation can take fifteen to twenty years. The segmented cactus looks like a green muffin; it is about six inches in length and two inches in diameter and is often topped by sprouting tufts of thick grayish-white hair. (Its genus name, *Lophophora*, means "I have tufts.") At certain times of year, a pink flower blooms.

Peyote is rich in plant alkaloids—at least fifty have been identified—but mescaline is the primary alkaloid in both peyote and San Pedro (huachuma) cactus.

**Also known as:** *Piote, hikuli, hikuri,* devil root, *challote,* cactus pudding, mescal button, *peote,* earth cactus, whiskey cactus.

---

* The epigraph comes from the title of French pharmacist Alexandre Rouhier's 1926 monograph.

**Active ingredients:** Mescaline, along with dozens of other alkaloids.

**Source:** Peyote cactus.

**Drug classification:** Serotonergic hallucinogen; phenethylamine.

**Methods of administration:** Oral ingestion, pulverized buttons, tea.

**Duration:** 8–14 hours.

**Open critical period:** Untested, estimated 3 weeks based on duration of journey.

### RISKS AND ADVERSE EFFECTS

There is no documented physical danger of eating high doses of peyote. Schultes reported seeing as many as ninety buttons eaten with no ill effects.[1] Low doses (fewer than four peyote buttons) produce no discernible effects in most people.

Peyote is not thought to create physical dependence. A 2005 study found no evidence of long-term neuropsychological deficits in members of the NAC, noting that these results may be context-dependent and not true for "illicit" use.[2] A similar conclusion was reached in a four-year,[3] large-scale study from

1971 on Navajo who regularly ate peyote, on average thirty-plus times per year. Among the Navajo there has been only one reported case where peyote, when used alone, was associated with a psychotic break; however, other reported psychotic episodes occurred when people with substance abuse or mental health problems used peyote.

### CONDITIONS ADDRESSED

Participants in peyote ceremonies report reductions in chronic anxiety, heightened community satisfaction, and increased sense of personal worth.[4] Some communities of the Native American Church use peyote to treat addiction to alcohol and other substances.

### DOSING GUIDELINES

Peyote is typically administered in ceremonies, the nature of which vary depending on the tradition they are associated with. Almost all are held at night, as peyote increases sensitivity to light, and they last until dawn. In ceremony, 30 to 150 grams of dry, pulverized peyote per person is typically ingested, the equivalent of six to twelve cactus buttons. Each button contains approximately 45 mg of mescaline.[5] The taste resembles exceedingly bitter green tea mixed with cement.

Sometimes a tea is prepared. One gram of powdered peyote tops (the equivalent of twelve to fifteen buttons) is reduced to twelve fluid ounces of tea.

> # Peyotists in the Native American Church say that the cactus, unlike alcohol, begins with the hangover first.[6]

### PROGRESSION OF A TYPICAL JOURNEY

Peyote is a long-acting psychedelic—a ceremony typically lasts twelve to fourteen hours. Effects have been described as more stimulating than psilocybin and less visionary than ayahuasca, but capable of inducing profound changes of perception, consciousness, and cognition. Colors (especially greens and violet) may be more vibrant; psychological insights, mystical experiences, and distortions in time, space, and self are common. One user reported seeing shadows that were disembodied from the objects casting them.

The alkaloids in the plant create a different set of subjective effects from pure mescaline. Peyote famously brings on synesthesia. It also has notable auditory effects. Natives say peyote brings them songs.

**Liftoff:** Begins about two hours after ingestion. Peyote typically induces nausea (and occasionally vomiting—one book about the drug was titled *The Miserable Miracle*), which ends after an hour. Purging is part of the process. It kick-starts the trip, during which most people feel an increase in emotional sensitivity or empathy. Visuals may begin and last for the next few hours.

**Comedown:** After six to twelve hours, effects gradually begin to diminish. It is usually difficult to sleep for at least twelve hours after ingestion because the plant's alkaloids are metabolized and excreted at different rates.

**Afterglow:** It's common to feel pleasantly relaxed, refreshed and at peace with the world, and hungry!

## HISTORY

Archaeologists in northeast Mexico and southern Texas have found peyote buttons dating back thousands of years. One sample was carbon-dated to around 3700 BCE.[7] Chemical analysis found that those buttons still contained 2 percent active mescaline, distinguishing them as the oldest psychoactive sample ever found.

In 1620, after the Spanish arrived in Mexico, they issued the Peyote Edict, which tried to ban peyote and all other plant medicines used by natives. Their brutal attempts at suppression went on for centuries, but natives continued to use peyote spiritually for rituals, healing, and divination and medicinally. One 1846 paper observed that people nibbled small doses several times a day as a tonic for the heart, perhaps history's first example of microdosing.

Peyote is still used by various tribes in Mexico. In the US, it is a legal sacrament used in ceremonies conducted by the Native American Church. The NAC combines different traditional beliefs with some elements of Christianity; its three hundred members constitute the largest indigenous religion in North America. NAC members use peyote at varying rates, between once per year and two to three times per week.[8] They guard their sacrament closely to protect it from outside interference and exploitation. However, the Global Drug Survey of 2017 doesn't even list peyote or mescaline among the forty most popular substances consumed.[9]

In Mexico, the worldview of the Wixárika people (also known as the Huichol) is intimately connected to peyote. The ceremonial calendar includes offerings, pilgrimages, festivals, and celebrations related to the knowledge bestowed by their sacred cactus.

One of their best-known rites is the pilgrimage to Wirikuta in the desert of San Luis de Potosí, during which pilgrims collect peyote for the celebrations that occur throughout the year. The Wixárika traditionally traveled the 250-mile route on foot under the blazing sun; today vehicles carry busloads of spiritual tourists, but the crowds have increased demand for peyote, further straining the species' survival.

# "Peyote is not for play.
# It is not for profit.
# It is not for everyone."

—Native American wisdom on how to get along with peyote

In 1936, twenty-one-year-old Richard Evans Schultes, then an anthropology student at Harvard, drove to Oklahoma to investigate peyote use among the Kiowa tribe.* Over the course of that summer, Schultes visited fifteen tribes and drank peyote with them two or three times a week. Though impressed by the kaleidoscopic visions the plant offered, he concluded that peyote's primary use was not to induce visions but rather as a universal remedy. One Kickapoo man told him that natives use peyote "as a white man uses aspirin." Other tribal contacts assured him that peyote used correctly renders other medicines unnecessary. The word for "medicine" is the same as for "peyote" in many tribal languages, with good reason according to modern chemical analysis.

## TRADITIONAL MEDICINAL USES

Peyote and San Pedro cactuses contain the alkaloids hordenine (peyocactin) and tyramine, both of which have antiseptic properties. For millennia, the Huichol have rubbed the juice of crushed peyote into wounds to prevent infection and promote healing. Hordenine has been shown to inhibit at least eighteen strains of penicillin-resistant *Staphylococcus* bacteria. It is also used to treat influenza, arthritis (rubbed on the skin to ease joint pain), tuberculosis, diabetes, intestinal disorders, snake and scorpion bites, and *Datura* poisoning. It has been reported to help poor eyesight—nearsightedness and astigmatism—and even blindness.

The Tarahumara people of northern Mexico consume small quantities of peyote to combat hunger, thirst, and exhaustion while on their long hunts. With peyote, it is said they can chase a deer for days without food, water, or rest.

Some Huichols use peyote to heal the planet. They travel to international festivals and conferences to make offerings to maintain alignment of the world's spiritual forces and to prevent them from being depleted. This is controversial among tribespeople. Some believe that taking this message to the wider world compromises sacred traditions; the counterargument is that navigating the space between tradition and modernity is crucial to the planet's survival.

---

* He described the peyote ceremonies he witnessed in two papers, "Peyote and Plants Used in the Peyote Ceremony" (1937) and "The Appeal of Peyote (*Lophophora williamsii*) as a Medicine" (1938).

## COULD PEYOTE ACHIEVE WORLD PEACE?

Margaret Mead had her suspicions . . .[10]

Pioneering anthropologist Margaret Mead came of age in the aftermath of World War I, as technologies like the radio and automobile began to radically change Western societies. She is most famous for her reports on the attitudes toward sex in indigenous South Pacific and Southeast Asian cultures; they were said to influence the 1960s sexual revolution. Less known were the utopian visions that she and her third husband, Gregory Bateson, formed based on peyote.

In the 1930s, while Mead was conducting fieldwork on the Omaha Reservation in Nebraska, she noticed that native people used peyote ritually to respond to social stresses and to promote social cohesion. "Rather than seeing peyote use among the Omaha as something which predates the modern era and goes back to an ancient tradition, Mead came to see it as something which was modern," Benjamin Breen, author of *Tripping on Utopia*, told NPR. "And it allowed people—and not just the Omaha, but potentially people in the rest of the world—to cope with the rapid technological changes they were going through." Mead's fascination with visionary substances was not a passing fascination. In 1954, she studied LSD as a tool to help humanity design peaceful, culturally diverse societies full of self-actualized individuals—in essence, a utopia.

If Mead were alive today and studying societal response to artificial intelligence, climate change, and social media run amok, I suspect she would view the psychedelic renaissance as a response to the same yearning for social cohesion and stress reduction the world was facing a century ago.

## THE US VERSUS PEYOTE: THE 150-YEAR WAR

The American Indian Religious Freedom Act Amendments of 1994 secured the right for over forty Native American nations to use peyote as a legal sacrament, but the battle was won at a deadly cost to their civilizations.

In 1845, US federal and state governments began suppressing peyote as part of a larger effort to annihilate and/or assimilate Native American cultures. The state of Texas force-marched all Native Americans to Oklahoma, sequestering them on "reservations" where they could be "managed." Many people died of starvation and cold in the ensuing years. The federal government then enacted "the Dance Ban," which aimed to quash all native

*CONTINUED*

celebrations as well as alcohol consumption. The Dance Ban failed to include peyote because the Feds didn't understand its importance to native cultures. Once the authorities realized peyote's integral role in native life, they classified the cactus as "alcohol" to enforce the ban.

In the early twentieth century, dozens of tribes came together to form a syncretic religion called the Native American Church (NAC). In the 1960s, the federal government again attempted to halt the religious use of the cactus, but the NAC fought the law for two decades until the Supreme Court legalized NAC sacramental use.

Peyote's place in native culture runs deeper than religion. "The peyote ceremony touches all aspects of native life," says Justin Jones, who is Navajo and provides general counsel to the NAC. It "really does give you that sense of identity, sense of belonging, sense of security. It's your culture, it's your identity, it's your language, it's your song. It's everything about you as an indigenous person." This is one reason indigenous people protect peyote and respect it as "a teacher to be listened to, not an object to investigate," wrote Mike Jay in his sweeping historical account, *Mescaline: A Global History of the First Psychedelic.*

In the 150-year war between the US government and peyote, the cactus won. But the battle continues on another front. Increased legal use in certain US cities is straining demand, while illegal poaching in combination with energy infrastructure projects (such as wind turbines and drilling) threatens the small selection of harvestable cactuses in the peyote gardens of southwestern Texas. The scarcity is worsened by mechanical plowing, which tears out the root along with the cactus, thus destroying the chance for new pups to grow.

The Indigenous Peyote Conservation Initiative (ipci.life) opened a nursery in 2022 in southern Texas to cultivate baby cacti in their native habitat. They hope to harvest two million pups a year, which can then be replanted on local ranches once they take hold. IPCI also has a distribution house where native peoples can go to access their medicine. As Steven S. Benally, an IPCI peyote conservationist and a Diné tribal member, told the *Guardian* in 2022, "Relying on some outsiders to take care of what our needs are—I think history has taught us that's never going to happen."[11]

# Mescaline: The Original Psychedelic

**Also known as:** Mescalito.

**Source:** Peyote cactus, San Pedro cactus, other cactus species, synthetic.

**Chemical name:** 3,4,5-trimethoxy-B-phenethylamine.

**Drug classification:** Serotonergic hallucinogen; phenethylamine. Like LSD, psilocybin, and DMT, mescaline is considered a classical psychedelic.

**Methods of administration:** Oral ingestion as a powder or in a capsule, or in dried cactus form.

**Duration:** 8–14 hours.

**Open critical period:** Untested, estimated 3 weeks based on duration.

## CONDITIONS ADDRESSED

Despite early promising reports decades ago, there is limited information about mescaline's potential as a therapeutic agent. A 2021 survey of adult users found that most people reported benefits in conditions including depression, anxiety, PTSD, and alcohol and drug use disorders.[12]

## DOSING GUIDELINES[13]

An active dose of oral mescaline sulfate is 150 to 800-plus mg. A common dosing suggestion is 3.75 mg mescaline per gram of body weight (1.7 mg/lb). Dose ranges are approximate and depend on individual sensitivity.

Threshold dose: 50–100 mg
Low dose: 100–200 mg
Average dose: 200–300 mg

High dose: 300–500 mg. This dose will spark intense visuals and possible ego dissolution—"an entheogenic all day lollipop" as described by one enthusiast who has posted in the erowid.org psychedelic experience libraries.

Heroic dose: 500–800-plus mg. This dose is for experienced users only.

## PROGRESSION OF A TYPICAL JOURNEY

The phases of a mescaline journey are similar to peyote but involve less nausea and fewer physical sensations. The effects of San Pedro are qualitatively different—see page 127.

## HISTORY

Considered the original psychedelic, mescaline is the naturally occurring phenethylamine* found in the peyote and Huachuma cacti. It was first isolated from peyote in 1897 by German chemist Arthur Heffter. He tried mescaline in various strengths on himself and noted that its effects were indistinguishable from peyote's.

When first identified, mescaline received a flurry of interest from European neurologists. The experiments they conducted spoke of dazzling visions, bizarre sensations, and cosmic revelations. Avant-garde painters worked under its influence, and clinicians administered it to philosophers including Jean-Paul Sartre and Walter Benjamin. Once LSD arrived in the 1940s, its shorter onset and fewer side effects stole mescaline's thunder as the mind-altering drug of choice.

Mescaline made a comeback in May 1953 when Humphry Osmond gave Aldous Huxley 400 grams of mescaline at his home in the

---

* Other substances in the phenethylamine group include MDA and MDMA, the neurotransmitters dopamine and adrenaline, and medications including antidepressants and bronchodilators.

## IS MDMA MESCALINE FOR THE INSTA GENERATION?

It's probably no accident that the uplifting feelings associated with mescaline resemble those of Ecstasy.[15] Alexander Shulgin inaugurated his psychedelic life on 400 grams of mescaline sulfate in 1960. In 1976, he devised a quick method of synthesizing MDMA, a tamer trip for a new generation that was more pressed for time and yearning for ritual. Both MDMA and the peyote ceremony use rhythm and movement, and both involve intense group bonding to lift the spirits. But unlike peyote or mescaline highs, which can grind on for twelve hours, MDMA is over in six.

Hollywood Hills. "This is how one ought to see, how things really are," Huxley recounted the following year in *The Doors of Perception*, which instantly became the canonical psychedelic text of the era. Every object in Huxley's vision was "all but quivering under the pressure of the significance with which they were charged,"[14] he wrote, describing realms that until that point had only been reserved for mystics and a handful of artists. He also introduced the metaphor of the brain as a "reducing valve" of consciousness that allows in only a fraction of the sensory awareness that we need to survive.

*The Doors of Perception* liberated psychedelic experimentation from the confines of scientific research and brought it into the open. William Burroughs, Allen Ginsberg, and Ken Kesey took inspiration from it. Jim Morrison named his band after the title. The book extolled mescaline all the way to its very last sentence: "*The man who comes back through the door in a wall will never be quite the same as the man who went out. He will be wiser, but less cocksure. Happier, but less self-satisfied. Humbler in acknowledging his ignorance yet better equipped to understand the relationship of words to things, of systematic reasoning to the unfathomable mystery which it tries forever vainly to comprehend.*"

By 1963, mescaline's uses were tightly controlled; it was placed into Schedule 1 shortly thereafter.

Mescaline can still be found on the dark web, but as author Mike Jay put it: "In the current psychedelic renaissance, the original psychedelic is conspicuous by its absence."[16]

## San Pedro, aka Huachuma, "The Plant That Awakens"

The San Pedro cactus is native to southern Ecuador, Peru, Chile, Bolivia, and Argentina at high altitudes, but it is cultivated throughout the Americas. Unlike peyote, it is tall, cylindrical, and quick growing. The strongest concentration of mescaline is found in the outer half inch of skin, where it serves as a parasite repellent. Mescaline makes up 0.053 to 4.7 percent of the whole fresh plant material by weight; this concentration is far less dense than peyote, which is why much more is required to achieve a psychedelic dose.[17] The more potent varieties are used in shamanic rituals.

Whereas peyote is small and difficult to see, San Pedro grows tall in a group of winding stems that fan proudly upward like organ pipes. The exterior skin ranges from dusty olive green to bright emerald, its thorns short and sparsely scattered. In spring, San Pedro blooms; the flower is closed during the day, but in early evening it opens into a single white-and-yellow bloom that emits a lemony scent. It is said that the San Pedro ceremony makes the participants' lives open like the night-blooming *Trichocereus* itself.

**Also known as:** *Achuma* (Bolivia) *aguacolla* and *gigantón* (Ecuador), Cactus of the Four Winds, the grandfather.

**Active ingredients:** Mescaline is the primary alkaloid of San Pedro; hordenine, lophophine, DMPEA (3,4-dimethoxyphenethylamine), and lobivine have also been detected.

**Source:** San Pedro cactus.

**Drug classification:** Mescaline, along with dozens of other alkaloids.

**Scientific name:** *Echinopsis* (also *Trichocereus*) *pachanoi.*

**Methods of administration:** Oral ingestion, pulverized cactus powder, tea.

**Duration:** 8–14 hours.

**Open critical period:** Untested, estimated 3 weeks based on duration.

### RISKS AND SIDE EFFECTS

The effects of San Pedro are similar to mescaline or peyote, but difficult experiences can occur, including anxiety, distress, confusion, paranoia, dizziness, and purging.

Amanda Elo'Esh, a California-based shaman trained in the Medicine Path Native American tradition, adds that huachuma is particularly tolerant and forgiving, especially compared with peyote's "warrior spirit." Her tradition calls it "the medicine of limitless and unconditional joy." That may be the case, but one thing is certain: There is little joy in the taste of the "yellow-green goo," which falls somewhere on the "Terrible to Disgusting" scale, and which is an unavoidable aspect of the experience.

### CONDITIONS ADDRESSED

Similar to peyote and mescaline, though it has been studied less.

### DOSING GUIDELINES

The concentration of active alkaloids varies widely among specimens. Potency testing for San Pedro and its many varieties is beyond the scope of this book.

Unlike peyote the flesh of which can be eaten, huachuma must be boiled and reduced until it is a dark yellow-green liquid with a mucus-like consistency that is intensely bitter. Sugar and lime are often added to the brew to blunt the bitterness and ginger chews can be used to sweeten the aftertaste.

As a rough guide a dose is typically one piece of cactus stalk, three to four inches in diameter.

- Twelve inches long for a plant of average potency
- Eighteen inches long for a weak variety
- Less than twelve inches long for a high-potency specimen

### PROGRESSION OF A TYPICAL SAN PEDRO JOURNEY

The different alkaloids in San Pedro produce a trip that is generally described as warmer or more mellow than peyote. Like peyote, it can last eight to fourteen hours.

It can take two to three hours for the full effects of San Pedro to be felt. The experience builds in waves. While deep introspection and confusion can occur, the trip is often described as energizing and remarkably lucid. Some users report it magnifies natural elements and has a "kind energy" likened to that of a grandfather.

A more descriptive take on San Pedro comes, as follows, from a contributor to Erowid, the world's largest repository of psychedelic experience. But remember, effects vary widely from person to person, plant to plant, setting to setting:

**Liftoff:** "The first noticeable effect is a slight dizziness, not at all disorienting like alcohol, but a barely perceptible lightness . . . "

**Peak:** "As if hit by a gust of wind, a great vision, a sharpening of the senses, a precise, crystal clearness of thought. A slowly spreading numbness flows through your body, a feeling of tranquility, so rare a treat in one's busy life. Next comes an eerie sort of detachment from our predictable, casual world. A visual force, a power, overwhelms us. All of our senses— seeing, hearing, tasting, smelling, touching— are linked to the others. A flood of perceptions being sucked in, through our eyes. One develops a sort of telepathic sense, the ability to transcend time, distance, and space, simply by envisioning it. The ability to discern and analyze every problem, and the lucidity to overcome it."

**Comedown**: Similar to peyote or mescaline.

## HISTORY

Fossils of San Pedro were found in Peru, in the Guitarrero cave of the Callejón de Huaylas valley, dating from 6800 to 6200 BCE, making it one of the oldest ancestral psychoactive plants. At the Chavín de Huántar site, also in Peru, stone engravings of San Pedro have been found along with textiles and ceramics. These objects date from the year 1300 BCE.

San Pedro was widely used in Peru when the Spaniards arrived. The Catholic Church slaughtered natives who took the drink, saying that it "deprives them of their senses and they see visions that the devil represents to them."[18] Native peoples renamed huachuma "San Pedro" after Peter, the Catholic saint, to give them cover from the murderous missionaries. (They chose the correct protector: In Catholicism, Peter holds the keys to heaven, a role "suggestive of the plant's power to open the gates between the visible and invisible worlds, allowing passage into the ecstatic realms."[19])

San Pedro is called the Cactus of the Four Winds because it has four ribs. It is collected near sacred lagoons high in the Andes and is typically harvested in late afternoon, when it is sweetest. The plant is considered a protector of families, marriage, and peaceful coexistence among family members, and is often cultivated close to homes. Healers use it diagnostically: They ingest San Pedro to "see" the nature of the patient's illness.

San Pedro can also be encountered in gardens and front yards everywhere from California to Goa to Thailand.[20] It is legal to grow San Pedro, but once it is harvested and made into tea, it becomes an illegal Schedule 1 substance in the US, Canada, Australia, and most of Europe (Spain and Portugal excepted).[21]

There are countless methods of growing and preparing huachuma. In the Andes, stalks of huachuma are commonly sold in markets sliced like bread and boiled for approximately seven hours in water. San Pedro may be taken alone or combined with other plants. The dried cactus powder can also be eaten if you have the stomach for it.

# IBOGAINE/IBOGA

## THE EVEREST OF PSYCHEDELICS

---

Ibogaine contributed much more than a reset of my neurochemistry...
I went from being unable to *not* take an opiate to feeling a very strong desire
to never use an opiate again. More important... I found a new-found
passion for pursuing a life of meaning and growth.[1]

TALIA EISENBERG, *cofounder, Beond Ibogaine Treatment Center*

Ibogaine is the least understood and longest-acting psychedelic. Early research has shown that a single treatment can eliminate withdrawal symptoms from opioids, cocaine, stimulants, alcohol, and nicotine; it can also diminish cravings for weeks, months, and sometimes years after administration. No other medicine does that. In high doses, it is thought to be one of the most powerful anti-addictive substances known and is a promising long-term addiction treatment. Some researchers theorize that it reverses the underlying brain disease that is at the heart of addiction.

Ibogaine is the synthesized alkaloid of the root bark of the plant *Tabernanthe iboga*, which grows in West Africa. Iboga (the Tsogho word for "to heal") is used as a sacrament for followers of the Bwiti cultural tradition in Gabon, Equatorial Guinea, and southern Cameroon. Iboga ceremonies can last for days; some stretch on for a week. They are considered healing rites for grief, jealousy, inner misdirection, and, more recently, as opioids have become a worldwide scourge, addiction and withdrawal. In Gabon, iboga itself is often referred to not as a plant but as a person or a being who connects humans to ancestors in the spirit world. This ancient construct is similar to South American plant medicines—even though the people on these two continents had no way of communicating until the last century.

**Also known as:** Iboga, the Addiction Interrupter.

**Source:** Primarily *Tabernanthe iboga*, also found in *Voacanga africana* and *Tabernaemontana undulata*.

**Chemical name:** 12-methoxyibogamine.

**Drug classification:** Serotonergic hallucinogen; tryptamine. Ibogaine has a highly complex pharmacology, interacting with many non-serotonergic targets in the brain, notably delta, kappa, and mu opioid receptors.

**Methods of administration:** In ceremony, iboga root bark is swallowed as a dry powder; it is less frequently served as a tea. In medical settings, ibogaine is administered as a series of pills.

**Duration:** 36–72 hours.

**Open critical period:** ~4+ weeks.

## CONDITIONS ADDRESSED

In the West, ibogaine is most commonly used for opioid use disorder and increasingly for addiction to fentanyl, a drug that is fifty times as powerful as heroin and kills the equivalent of a planeload of people a day in the US alone. Unlike other substance abuse medicines (Suboxone, buprenorphine, methadone), which have limited effectiveness,* small studies demonstrate that ibogaine stops withdrawal symtoms immediately, reduces cravings, and contributes to long-term cessation.[2] Some addicts report never using again.

It also helps lower the depression that accompanies withdrawal; more than a few addicts claim it guides them to "their purpose" and redirects the course of their lives. That may sound like New Age magical thinking, but Dr. Deborah Mash, professor of neurology and of molecular and cellular pharmacology at the University of Miami and CEO of the drug company DemeRx, has researched ibogaine since 1992. She says it activates a "today I've switched gears" effect in the brain.[3]

When it comes to addiction, withdrawal and relapse are two different things. As far as relapse is concerned, one small study in the US and New Zealand showed that one-third to one-half of the subjects treated with ibogaine do not return to using.[4] This is the same efficacy as methadone, the difference being that ibogaine achieved those results with one dose versus lifelong maintenance. Nor does ibogaine lead to cravings for more ibogaine, although some patients return for a maintenance dose if or when the effects begin to wear off.

Beond, an ibogaine treatment center in Cancun, Mexico, claims that ibogaine can stanch other behaviorally driven conditions including gambling addiction, eating disorders, and the newly coined CUD, cellphone use disorder.

### Traumatic Brain Injury (TBI)

In one 2024 observational study supported by VETS** (Veterans Exploring Treatment Solutions), thirty US special operations veterans with head trauma, combat exposure, or blast exposure received ibogaine treatment in conjunction with therapy at the Ambio Life Sciences clinic in Mexico.[5] One month following treatment, the vets reported that their TBI symptoms went from "moderate disability" to "no disability." Suicidal ideation decreased from 47 percent to 7 percent. PTSD, anxiety, and depression were all reduced, and cognitive function improved. No serious side effects or heart complications were reported. Worth noting is that these veterans were also engaged in complementary treatments (therapy, coaching, group activities) while at the clinic, which may have contributed substantially to the positive outcomes.

Dr. Nolan Williams, associate professor of psychiatry and behavioral sciences and the director of the Brain Stimulation Lab at Stanford, called the results of that study "dramatic." The board of scientists who reviewed

---

* According to Dr. Kenneth Alper, the most widely cited researcher on the topic, "Only a fraction of those with Opioid Use Disorder access medical assisted therapy. When they do, one-third or more will drop out within eight months. Mean lengths of stay in treatment is on the order of six to eight months. While in treatment use of illicit opioids is 20–60 percent. Completion of detox fails a third to half of the time." From "Kentucky Opioid Abatement Commission Public Hearing," 2023.

** Founded in 2019, Veterans Exploring Treatment Solutions (VETS) is a 501(c)(3) nonprofit organization working to end veteran suicides by providing resources, research, and advocacy for US military veterans seeking psychedelic-assisted therapies primarily for traumatic brain injury (TBI), post-traumatic stress disorder (PTSD), and addiction.

"**I went from being constantly angry and feeling alone, burdened by the trauma of war and the loss of twelve friends to suicide, to finding a renewed sense of hope and peace. The turning point was ibogaine treatment. Today, I am grateful to sleep well, live without daily fight or flight reactions, and look forward to life with newfound hope.**"[6]

—PATRICK FLATLEY,
US Army Green Beret veteran
and ibogaine study participant

the study, none of whom are known for their hyperbolic enthusiasm, pronounced the results "striking."

### Other Uses for Ibogaine

Theoretical papers and a few anecdotal cases have suggested that small doses of ibogaine may be effective in reducing symptoms of Parkinson's disease, a condition that affects an estimated seven to ten million people worldwide.[7]

A small but growing number of entrepreneurs are heading to ibogaine clinics for what they're calling "psychospiritual tune-ups," though there doesn't seem to be any universally accepted understanding of what a "tune-up" entails.

Other groups are experimenting with ibogaine microdosing for people who are not addicts and who have no existing medical issues. One organization, IbogaQuest, located in Tepoztlán, Mexico, has developed an eight-week iboga microdosing regimen that costs about $800, medicine included.

This is supported by meditation, journaling, and two hours of online weekly group therapy. "The experience is very grounding," says Vincente Alonso, a psychologist and the lead therapist of IbogaQuest. "Like meditation iboga can give you the same sort of distance between what's going on inside and watching how you react. But a lot of the healing happens in the relationships established in the group. When you hear other people struggling with things similar to yours, it lessens the isolation you may be feeling. The whole program is like a balm to the heart."

Whereas microdosing psilocybin can feel emotionally opening, and LSD is said to provide more of an energizing lift, microdosing iboga is

"LSD is like a look out of a window into the open; ibogaine is more like an occasion to destroy the old building and make room for a new one. It is more of a 'work drug' in the sense of facilitating an analytical process on the unconscious obstacles to life."

—CHILEAN PSYCHIATRIST
CLAUDIO NARANJO,
*The Healing Journey*

described as more clarifying. "I think of it like a truth serum," adds another iboga microdosing guide, Kristie Jacobsen, founder of Casa-Well, also located in Tepoztlán. "It's a bit more confrontational and clarifying."

**Adverse effects:** It is still unclear, given ibogaine's relative newness in the West, if microdosing ibogaine carries the same cardiac risks as a full flood dose. Those with a heart condition should not experiment with this drug until more research is conducted. IbogaQuest has had no reported adverse reactions in the few years it has been running microdosing programs. Another interesting factor to consider: There were no reported adverse effects in France from 1930 to 1966, when Lambarène, a low-dose ibogaine-derived "tonic," was sold legally throughout the country. It's very possible the adverse effects are dose-dependent, but we will not know conclusively until more research and trials are run.

## DOSING GUIDELINES
### Flood dose

8–15 mg/kg (3.6–6.8 mg/lb).[8] This is the therapeutic detox dose.

### Psychospiritual tune-up dose

13 mg/kg (5.9 mg/lb).

### Maintenance dose

100–300 mg doses are offered if drug cravings recur; this dose is thought to extend the exposure to noribogaine, the metabolite* that curtails withdrawal symptoms.

### Low dose

Low doses (also called hunter's doses in Gabon) are less disruptive and are described as pleasant, great for walking around, and sometimes sexually stimulating. In Central Africa, a small amount of iboga root is commonly

---

* A metabolite is a by-product that occurs after the body breaks down food, drugs, or chemicals.

mixed with cannabis and smoked for a pleasant afternoon sojourn.

### Microdose

There are no established protocols. IbogaQuest starts people at 200 mgs and escalates over eight weeks. A significant difference between microdosing ibogaine and other psychedelics is that iboga/ibogaine is converted to noribogaine in the liver, which keeps it in the system for a long time, creating a cumulative effect.

## PROGRESSION
## OF A TYPICAL CLINICAL JOURNEY

When used clinically for the treatment of addiction, ibogaine hydrochloride, a purified version of the root bark, is administered in gelcaps, typically in three doses.

**Test dose:** The first administration serves as a "test dose," administered two hours prior to the flood dose. During this period, a patient's heart rate, allergic response, and vital signs are monitored to ensure no complications arise.

**Flood dose:** Once safety is established, the person is given two more capsules over three hours. Once this dose fully hits the bloodstream, withdrawal symptoms dissolve almost immediately.

**Acute stimulation phase:** The first four to six hours of the "acute stimulation phase" can be visual and psychedelic, something akin to an intense lucid dream. During this phase, patients lie down, close their eyes, and turn inward. There may be nausea, vomiting, or ataxia (loss of balance or the ability to stand). Unlike any other psychedelic, ibogaine induces what is frequently described as a "life review" or a cathartic replay of important memories.

**Peak:** Once maximum concentrations peak, visuals cease (in fact, visions stop anytime eyes

open) and subjects enter a state of deep introspection in which they revisit past fears or traumas without the associated emotional charge. Sometimes a path to change is laid out for them. Not only have patients reported improvements in brain injuries, but they "became observers of their own life experience," says Stanford's Williams. "You are able to forgive, forget or understand another person's position as well as your own and seemingly unlock the lock on both sides and dissolve the problem. [Patients] had a pronounced cathartic reevaluation—reconsolidation—of past life problematic memories."[9]

**Landing, aka the Gray Day:** "Twenty-four hours later, once patients are down the slide, they are in the wading pool of recovery," says Jonathan Dickinson, CEO of Ambio Life Sciences, who has administered over a thousand ibogaine treatments. Most people sleep through the night and wake up feeling better, if not refreshed.

**Post-treatment:** After a journey, a person remains in care for an additional ten to fourteen days, undergoing psychological integration, therapy, and monitoring. Some return for follow-up treatments. Others are one and done.

### RISKS AND ADVERSE EFFECTS

More than ten thousand people have been treated with ibogaine to date, mostly in countries where it is unregulated.[10] Known side effects during treatment include dizziness, confusion, and ataxia, which is sometimes followed by nausea or vomiting. But the biggest concern with ibogaine are the thirty-three known deaths associated with its use. That is an alarmingly high number that has stood in the way of wider clinical acceptance.

> "I call iboga the washing machine. It starts talking to you, like 'You rotten motherfucker. You said *that,* you haven't paid that bill, you did that terrible thing,' and it's going around and around in your head. And then it starts to go down your belly and then to your heart, and then ... well ... 'Maybe you're not so bad,' and then you hit the rinse cycle and it spins it all out of you and you're feeling great."

—DIMITRI MUGIANIS,
Cardea cofounder and one of the first ibogaine providers in the West

Ibogaine is known to extend the QT interval of the heartbeat, the span of time it takes the heart to contract and refill with blood before it beats again. This puts people with heart conditions at risk for life-threatening arrhythmia. A 2012 paper by Dr. Kenneth Alper examined autopsies of nineteen people who died in ibogaine treatment and found that the deaths were caused by preexisting heart conditions, impure ibogaine (probably purchased on the gray market, where quality is uncontrolled), excessive doses, or the presence of other drugs in the system, including opioids, either while the person was undergoing the treatment or shortly after. Overall, he concluded that there is no clear evidence that pure ibogaine or iboga itself causes heart attack, cardiac arrest, or arrhythmia.[11]

However, the jury is still very much out on ibogaine's safety profile. Warnings should be heeded.

*Warning:* People with heart conditions are at risk for life-threatening arrhythmia when taking ibogaine.

*Warning:* Until robust research is conducted, people with any heart condition or who are severely obese should not take ibogaine before consulting with their doctors. They should also be sure that any facility they enter is staffed with qualified medical and post-treatment care staff.

*Warning:* Certain people, mostly women, are also predisposed to have mutations in the CYP2D6 enzyme and metabolize ibogaine poorly.* When ibogaine is metabolized more slowly, it can build up in the body, reaching

* CYP2D6 is a gene that metabolizes many antidepressant and antipsychotic medications. The mutation can be determined by genetic testing.

dangerous levels. For these people, dosing must be adjusted accordingly. In any case, consuming quinine, grapefruit, and any food that is metabolized by the CYP2D6 enzyme should be avoided before treatment, as they can also increase cardiac risks.

*Warning:* Adverse interactions may also occur between ibogaine and some psychiatric medications. When ibogaine is used for addiction, the patient's drug of choice should be completely cleared from the body before and during treatment.[12] Opioids, as an example, are also metabolized by CYP2D6 and will compete with ibogaine for a place in line. This can lead to dangerous buildups of either or both in the body.

## HOW DOES IBOGAINE TREAT ADDICTION?

How ibogaine works to curtail addiction and limit withdrawal symptoms is still a mystery. But here's what we do know: Heroin addicts need increasing amounts of heroin because their bodies quickly build a tolerance to the opioid. The body reduces its production of endorphins, and the amounts it does produce are insufficient to meet the demand. When this occurs, withdrawal begins; addicts feel cravings or depression, which are only relieved by more opioids or methadone. Any sort of depression or disturbing event can trigger a relapse.

Ibogaine appears to work differently. Once in the system, ibogaine/iboga is converted by the liver to its metabolite noribogaine. Noribogaine stays in the body for several weeks after treatment and diminishes or eliminates the cravings and depression that follow with-drawal. Mood stays elevated and cravings remain low, giving patients the physical and emotional space to complete a transition to abstinence.

Pharmacologically, ibogaine also appears to affect an abundance of neurotransmitters, including opioid, serotonin, dopamine, NMDA glutamate, and nicotinic acetylcholine. It also seems to reduce cravings for cocaine and nicotine.

Some, but not all, patients require follow-up dosing, which can be undertaken at three-month intervals.

## HISTORY

Archaeological evidence indicates that indigenous people in Gabon have been using iboga for at least two thousand years. Legend has it that Pygmies stumbled upon iboga's psychoactive effects after observing animals nibbling the *Tabernanthe iboga* plant. The Pygmies shared what they learned with Bantu people, who make up the majority of Gabon's population.

French and Belgian explorers in the nineteenth century first described the stimulant and aphrodisiac effects of eating iboga root. In 1901, French pharmacologists isolated ibogaine. In the 1930s, an antidepressant and stimulant tonic, Lambarene, was bottled and marketed in France. Sales continued until 1966, when the French government outlawed it along with all other ibogaine products in response to the incipient War on Drugs.

Prior to this, in 1962, Howard Lotsof, a nineteen-year-old American heroin user, was given ibogaine by a chemist friend. After one dose that lasted a whopping thirty-three hours, his drug cravings stopped. Lotsof spent the rest of his life lobbying independent researchers, pharmaceutical companies, the NIH, and NIDA to test ibogaine as a treatment for heroin addiction. In 1993, the FDA approved a Phase I clinical trial, but it was abruptly halted due to contractual and financial disputes between Lotsof and the investigators running the trial.

Today, as opioid addiction has escalated into a global crisis with no new anti-addiction medicines on the horizon, legal ibogaine treatment centers have sprung up in New Zealand, South Africa, and the state of São Paulo in Brazil. There are iboga treatment centers in Mexico, Costa Rica, Panama, the Netherlands, and Portugal, where it is neither illegal nor regulated. Health Canada added ibogaine to its Prescription Drug List in 2017, but it is still not available for treatment.

Inpatient treatment typically lasts two weeks and costs $15,000 to $20,000.

Drug companies including MindMed, Delix, and Gilgamesh are investigating analogs that mimic ibogaine's anti-abuse properties with a safer profile, shorter mechanisms of action, and no hallucinations. Skeptics say ibogaine without visions is like wine without alcohol—the visions are key to healing and learning—but time will tell. These novel compounds are in early-stage development.

## THE IBOGA CEREMONY

The iboga ceremony is an integral part of the Bwiti tradition in Gabon and southern Cameroon. Bwiti has been described as something between a religion and a shamanic tradition of the forest people of the Central African rainforest. About 5 percent of the population engages in these communal ceremonies, which often run for days and involve elaborate costumes, music, and colorful makeup.

During the ceremony, the shaved root of the iboga plant (also called *bois sacre* or sacred wood) is swallowed as a powder in great quantities, sometimes as many as thirty-six tablespoons over the course of several hours, and washed down with water.* The bark's texture is akin to sawdust, and the taste is described as disgustingly bitter—several iboga users I interviewed visibly squirmed when they recalled swallowing it.

Once iboga takes hold, initiates become *baanzi*, "one who has seen the other world." They lie down for hours while community members support them by playing instruments, chanting, and singing. Community members of all ages, children included, may take a low dose that works as a stimulant without any psychedelic response. After the ceremony, initiates often bathe in water infused with other forest plants to cleanse their psyches of any threatening or harmful mental, emotional, or spiritual residue.

In 1999, the writer Daniel Pinchbeck went to Gabon to participate in an iboga ceremony. "It was one of the most difficult, yet rewarding, experiences of my life," he wrote in the *Guardian*.[13] "I had heard the substance described as 'Ten years of psychoanalysis in a single night' but, of course, I did not believe it.

"As the tribesmen played drums and sang around me until dawn, I lay on a concrete floor and journeyed back through the course of my life, witnessing forgotten scenes from childhood. At one point, I had a vision of a wooden statue walking across the room and sitting in front of me—later, I was told this was 'the spirit of iboga' coming out to communicate with me . . .

"The initiation, which lasted more than twenty hours, was ultimately liberating. I was shown my habitual overuse of alcohol and the effect it was having on my relationships, my

---

* There are two types of iboga ceremonies in Gabon. The *dissoumba* or turtle ceremony involves taking a massive dose of iboga and withdrawing deeply into your internal world. The presence of villagers remind baanzi that they are not alone. In the *missoko* or catfish ceremony, participants take a lower dose and the ceremony leader stays nearby questioning and talking to the baanzi.

# WHO WAS HOWARD LOTSOF?

In 1962, Howard Lotsof was a precocious film student hanging out on the post-Beat, pre-hippie Lower East Side of New York. He wore a pocket pen holder and suspenders—and presented as a hipster nerd long before it became a type. But he was also crafty enough to have formed a pharmaceutical company that allowed him to legally purchase morphine and cocaine. In short order he had developed a heroin habit that was spinning out of control.

One day a chemist friend was cleaning his freezer and gave Lotsof a large dose of ibogaine—which at the time was virtually unknown in the West. This set him off on a thirty-three-hour trip that included an hour-long session with his shrink and a vivid tour through his childhood memories. When it ended, he fell asleep thinking, "I'll never take this drug again," but when he awakened he realized he had spent the entire journey without going through withdrawal. He gave ibogaine to seven other addicts. Five stopped using immediately.

Lotsof spent the rest of his life advocating for ibogaine as a legal addiction treatment. He worked underground in Amsterdam and with mainstream scientists. In the mid-1980s, he persuaded a Belgian company to manufacture ibogaine in capsule form and begin offering it to addicts in the Netherlands. Of the thirty addicts he treated, twenty stopped using for periods ranging from four months to four years. He traveled to Gabon and somehow arranged a meeting with the president, Omar Bongo, who gifted him several pounds of root bark to take back to the West. "Iboga is Gabon's gift to the world," Bongo pronounced.[14]

With no advanced degree, Lotsof wrote over sixty scientific papers on ibogaine and lobbied world-class researchers and addiction recovery specialists to initiate clinical studies. "It took me from 1984 to 1991 through the leadership of three different directors of NIDA to finally get them to take a serious look at ibogaine," he said in a 2004 video made for ICEERS.[15] But there was tremendous resistance. "Imagine you're a doctor. You spend twelve years getting your education, you spend fifteen years . . . becoming an expert. The last thing you're going to want to hear is that some former heroin addict discovered the effective medicine you've been looking for."

Lotsof died at sixty-six in 2020 of liver cancer but remained resolute in his conviction that ibogaine "converts an addict on day one to a non-addict on day three."

writing, and my psyche. When I returned to the US, I steadily reduced my drinking to a fraction of its previous level—an adjustment that seems to be permanent."

## IBOGA AND SUSTAINABILITY

The growing demand for iboga has put a strain on the wild populations of the plant. Gabon declared iboga a "national treasure" in 2000 and in 2019 halted all exports in an attempt to force producers to follow the Nagoya Protocol. Nagoya was written to prevent exploitation by establishing benefit sharing for the people who live where healing plants originate.

The iboga plant takes two to four years to grow and only thrives in soil conditions found in equatorial jungles. Harvesting and replanting must be done sustainably to ensure crop regeneration. Gabon is a poor country of 2.3 million people with limited resources and infrastructure to enforce laws. At the moment there is a brisk illegal trade fueled by poachers from neighboring Cameroon, who cross the border to steal plants and sell processed iboga at inflated prices on the black market.

Blessings of the Forest (blessingsofthe-forest.org) is a nonprofit working to change that. Rather than planting trees, Blessings provides financial and technical support to locals to form associations and establish iboga plantations. It connects village associations with international buyers and helps with export paperwork. In return, communities agree not to cut down large shrubs and to reinvest at least half of what they earn from iboga sales into community projects such as schools and infrastructure.

Once this program is running smoothly, Blessings says its next priority is to convince—or, if necessary, legally obligate—ibogaine clinics and pharmaceutical companies around the world to engage in some form of reciprocity for Gabon. Without that, it's "biopiracy," according to Yann Guignon, Blessings' codirector.

Protecting iboga (and other natural sources of visionary medicines) is increasingly important now, as rising demand coupled with lax international regulation threatens to erode sustainable development. No plant can thrive if it is overharvested to the point of extinction.

# PSYCHEDELIC SUPPLEMENTS

## KAVA, KRATOM, KANNA, CACAO

--------------------------------------------------------

The following plant medicines are known to provoke gentle changes in consciousness; some can be combined with more powerful psychedelics to enhance or quietly alter the experience. They are legal, though unregulated, in most of the world and often considered "nutritional supplements" or "nutraceuticals."

Bear in mind that all plant medicines, regardless of their legal status, vary depending on the quality of the plants from which they are derived and their methods of processing. The best way to ensure quality is to look for products that have been tested for purity, pesticides, and residual solvents by an independent (or third-party) lab.

## Kava

Kava is a very well-studied mind- and mood-enhancing substance. It has been used throughout Oceania and the South Pacific long before history was recorded. First accounts date back to Captain Cook's second voyage to the South Pacific, 1772 to 1775.

Drinking kava can reportedly lead to tranquility; it is used to soothe anxiety, depression, and sleeplessness.

Kava is integral to life in the Oceania region, and it is essential to community gatherings and rituals. Virtually all visitors to the Oceania islands are served kava when they come.

**Chemistry:** Kava's mood-enhancing and relaxing effects are due to compounds called kavalactones, which act primarily as muscle relaxants. They interact with GABA A receptors, which contributes to Kava's calming and sedative qualities. They also inhibit the reuptake of norepinephrine and dopamine, which contribute to its mood-enhancing qualities.

Double-blind placebo-controlled studies conducted at Duke University have shown that while kava is a sedative, it does not impair mental function, memory, or clarity of thought, unlike prescription tranquilizers.[1]

**Method of administration:** Kava is a bitter-tasting tea or beverage made from the ground roots of the *Piper metysticum* plant, a leafy member of the pepper family.

**Adverse reactions:** The trials at Duke University show that kava is safe and somewhat effective at reducing situational anxiety (but not generalized anxiety disorder) and stress, but doesn't lead to physiological dependence or withdrawal. Another small study, also at Duke, suggested found it may reduce the risk of heart attack.

There are very few side effects at recommended doses, but when used to excess (the equivalent of drinking a gallon per day) it can lead to shortness of breath, dry skin, liver damage, alteration to white blood cells, and malnutrition. It is hard to imagine consuming this amount of kava on a daily basis.

There was a flurry of reports of kava causing liver damage when taken in an alcoholic extract, but no conclusive evidence was ever found. Avoid mixing kava with alcohol, especially if you have a history of liver damage or disease.

**Conditions addressed:** In addition to its sedative qualities, kava is used medicinally to treat urogenital inflammation and cystitis, to relieve headaches, restore vigor, soothe upset stomach, cure whooping cough in children, and ease symptoms of asthma and tuberculosis. Used topically, it treats fungal infections and soothes stings and skin inflammation.

**Dosing:** Researchers at Duke University Medical School found that 70 to 100 mgs of kava three times per day (or 210 to 280 mg daily) effectively treats anxiety. [2]

To promote sleep, take 140 to 210 mg of kava thirty to sixty minutes before bed.

**Home preparation**: Kava bars are in full swing in many cities, but it's easy to prepare the drink at home.

Place two to four tablespoons of kava root in a strainer bag or empty tea bag. This reduces the sediment buildup as it steeps.

Add eight to twelve ounces of warm, not hot, water. Squeeze or "knead" the kava powder as it steeps for about ten minutes. The water will turn densely brown.

Drink up!

*Note:* Kava is not delicious. It is generously described as "earthy," though I think "wet clay" or "mud" are more fitting descriptions. Some people add ginger, honey, lemon, or pumpkin spice to mask the bitter flavor. Milk or fatty nut milks like coconut or almond also help draw out kava's active constituents.

## Kratom

Kratom is a powder derived from the leaves of *Mitragyna speciosa*, a tree native to Southeast Asia and related to the coffee tree. Kratom is still used as a traditional medicine in Thailand, Indonesia, Malaysia, and Papua New Guinea. Lower doses are used to increase focus; higher doses as used as an analgesic to help relieve pain.

**Chemistry:** The leaves of *M. speciosa* contain over forty compounds. They interact with opioid receptors but also stimulate the serotonin and norepinephrine receptor systems, which may contribute to kratom's stimulating and mood-enhancing properties.

**Effects:** Just like cannabis, the effects of kratom vary depending on dose and strain. Lower doses produce mild caffeine-like effects (stimulation, sharper focus or motivation). Higher doses are more sedative and euphoric, less intense than opioids, and often described as warm, comforting, and contented. Depending on strain and dose, the stimulating and sedative effects may occur simultaneously, resulting in a pleasant state that is both energized and relaxed.

One Erowid contributor said a month of steady kratom use provided him with "a nice buzz, an obvious change in headspace, and all around was a pleasant way to get away from sobriety in a hedonistic way, while retaining my ability to not only do my job, but to do it well."[3]

**Adverse effects/abuse potential:** Kratom has low toxicity relative to dose. Fatal doses from kratom use alone are extremely rare. One reason kratom is said to be safer than/superior to other opioids is that it is not lethal at higher doses—you will vomit before you take enough to kill you.[4]

Moderate use of kratom is not known to create any long-term complications. However, given its mood-enhancing, pain-relieving qualities, some medical practitioners have raised concern about its potential for abuse. There are reports that regular, repeated use can become addictive and habit forming.

Use with caution if you have a tendency toward substance dependence.

**Side effects:** Loss of appetite, weight loss, constipation, decreased libido, apathy, anxiety, dizziness, headaches, heart palpitations, nausea.

**Conditions addressed:** Users claim kratom is helpful in weaning off opioids and methamphetamine, especially in the early stages of withdrawal.

**Dosing:** 0.025 g/lb for stimulation; 0.04 g/lb for pain relief and relaxation.

**Duration of effects:**[5] Onset: Ten to forty minutes.

**Journey:** Two to five hours.

**Comedown and aftereffects:** Up to twelve hours.

**Method of administration:** Fresh or dried leaves can be chewed, but the taste is quite bitter. Kratom is more often powdered, steeped in warm to hot (not boiling) water, and served as a tea, the acrid taste masked with honey or lemon juice. Other users prefer to mix powdered kratom in olive oil, since the fats in oil help mask the bitterness.

Avoid mixing kratom and magic mushrooms: Since mitragynine, an opioid alkaloid found in the plant, is a serotonin 2A antagonist and psilocin is a serotonin 2A agonist, kratom can counteract and decrease the pleasurable psychedelic effects of magic mushrooms. Combining them is not unsafe, but it may diminsh the journey.[6]

Legality: Kratom products are legal in the US and accessible online.

## Kanna

Kanna is a plant that grows in certain deserts of South Africa. Its fermented roots have been used medicinally by the San and Khoikhoi peoples for hundreds of years. It is primarily known as a sedative but can produce a variety of effects depending on the combination of its active ingredients.

**Also known as:** canna, channa, kaugoed (means "something to chew" in Dutch or Afrikaans).

**Source:** *Sceletium tortuosum*, a succulent ground cover that produces white flowers with thin petals.

**Drug classification:** Inebriating sedative.

**Effects:** Kanna has gained an international reputation due to its stress-reducing, empathogenic, and calming effects; modern plant medicine practitioners commonly refer to kanna as a heart opener in reference to its supposed empathogenic qualities. Some people use it as an alternative to alcohol.

An article on Vice.com once claimed that kanna was "MDMA-lite," a massive overstatement that of course sparked tons of interest.[7]

**Risks and adverse effects:** Used on its own, kanna is known to be a safe product. However, mixing it with MDMA, SSRIs, MAOIs, or 5-HTP could put you at risk for serotonin syndrome. For some people, the come-on can cause dizziness or slight nausea. These effects subside quickly and settle into a mellow, joyful headspace.

**Active ingredients:** The fermented roots and leaves of kanna contain twenty-eight active, mildly psychoactive alkaloids; mesembrine, mesembrenone, tortuosamine, and delta

7 mesembrenone are the main components. These compounds act similarly to SSRIs, which might explain kanna's mood-enhancing or joyful qualities.

**Methods of administration:** Oral ingestion (placed on the tongue or mixed into water or a smoothie) as a tea or tincture. Snorting (insufflation) delivers the most powerful hit.

**Conditions addressed:** Various studies show kanna is effective for reducing anxiety and depression; elevating mood; promoting relaxation, sleep, and endurance; and relieving hunger, abdominal pain, and toothache. Its compounds have also been used as antimicrobial, antioxidant, anti-inflammatory agents.

Kanna has been sold as the nutraceutical supplement Zembrin for some thirty years. Placebo-controlled double-blind trials show it can effectively reduce anxiety, but it is not a long-term solution.[8]

**Dosing:** Like all plant medicines, dosing depends on species, how you take it, and your own metabolism. For example, one brand, Kanna Extracts, produces two different varieties, each containing different ratios of three active alkaloids.

Lift has 85 percent mesembrine, 10 percent mesembrenone, and 5 percent delta 7 mesembrenone. This is said to produce energizing effects.

Bliss has 60 percent mesembrine, 20 percent mesembrenone, and 20 percent delta 7 mesembrenone. This is said to produces warm-hug, "melty" effects.

It's likely that additional kanna mixtures will be coming to market as the product grows in popularity.

**History:** The Khoikhoi and San peoples of South Africa have used kanna since ancient times as an essential part of their culture and pharmacopeia. Hunter-gatherers used it to increase the endurance needed for hunting and to manage the stress that comes with living in dry and challenging environments.[9]

## Cacao

Cacao are the beans of a small evergreen tree native to the tropical regions of Central and South America. Humans have been using cacao seeds (commonly known as cocoa beans) to make chocolate for thousands of years, but cacao is not the same as chocolate.

High-quality cacao is harvested from a specific type of *Theobroma cacao* tree called criollo. Criollo trees are less hardy and have a milder taste than the forastero variety used by the chocolate industry, but their fruit contains more of the mildly consciousness-altering compounds like theobromine and serotonin.

**Active ingredients:** Cacao is considered a superfood due to its high concentration of vitamins, minerals, and antioxidants. In its unrefined form, it contains 145 distinct compounds. The most pharmacologically significant are theobromine, phenylethylamine, anandamide, MAO, and tryptophan.

Theobromine* has an energizing effect without creating the jitters of coffee. Phenylethylamine releases the feel-good chemical dopamine. Anandamide works on cannabinoid receptors to create a feeling of euphoria (the name of the molecule comes from *ananda*, the Sanskrit word for "bliss"). Cacao also contains

---

* The word *theobroma* is from ancient Greek and means "food of the gods."

antioxidants and minerals including magnesium and iron.

**Risks and adverse effects:** Adverse effects usually occur in response to high doses (over 2 ounces, or 55 g) and include headache, dizziness or nausea, sleeplessness, anxiety, lightheadedness, or sweaty palms.

*Warning:* People with heart conditions or who are currently taking antidepressants or hypertension medications should tread lightly with cacao since theobromine can increase heart rate.

Theobromine is also toxic to dogs and cats, so store cacao out of their reach.

**Tolerance/dependence:** Chocolate can be habit forming, as chocoholics can attest, but hardly dangerous. Cacao's bitterness makes it less likely to be consumed habitually.

**Methods of administration:** Ceremonial cacao is served as a beverage.

**Preparation:** Grate or chop cacao paste and add this into gently heated water (not boiling). The common ratio is about 1 to 2 ounces (28 to 55 grams) of cacao per cup of water. Cinnamon, nutmeg, or other spices can be added to alter the taste.

**Benefits / conditions addressed:** Ceremonial cacao is served before a psilocybin journey.

The two have been ceremonial allies for hundreds of years in Central and South American traditions. Cacao is said to make some people more attuned to the expansive qualities of psychedelics.

Cacao has a very mild effect. It's "neuroactive but not strongly psychoactive," says James Giordano, professor of neurology and biochemistry at Georgetown University Medical Center.[10] Effects are described as warm and uplifting, alerting yet comforting, inspiring greater receptivity to one's feelings and vulnerabilities. Plant medicine people commonly refer to cacao as a heart opener. Physiologically at least, this is true, as it is a vasodilator and stimulates the cardiovascular system.

Cacao has been linked to health benefits including reduced inflammation, along with enhanced mood and cognitive function.

**Dosing guidelines:** A standard ceremonial dose is 40 to 50 grams (1.5 to 1.8 ounces) of shaved cacao paste. New users may want to start at half this amount and work their way up until they feel a sufficient reaction.

**History:** Cacao was first discovered by the Olmec people in early Mesoamerica and was used widely in rituals by the Aztecs and Mayans.

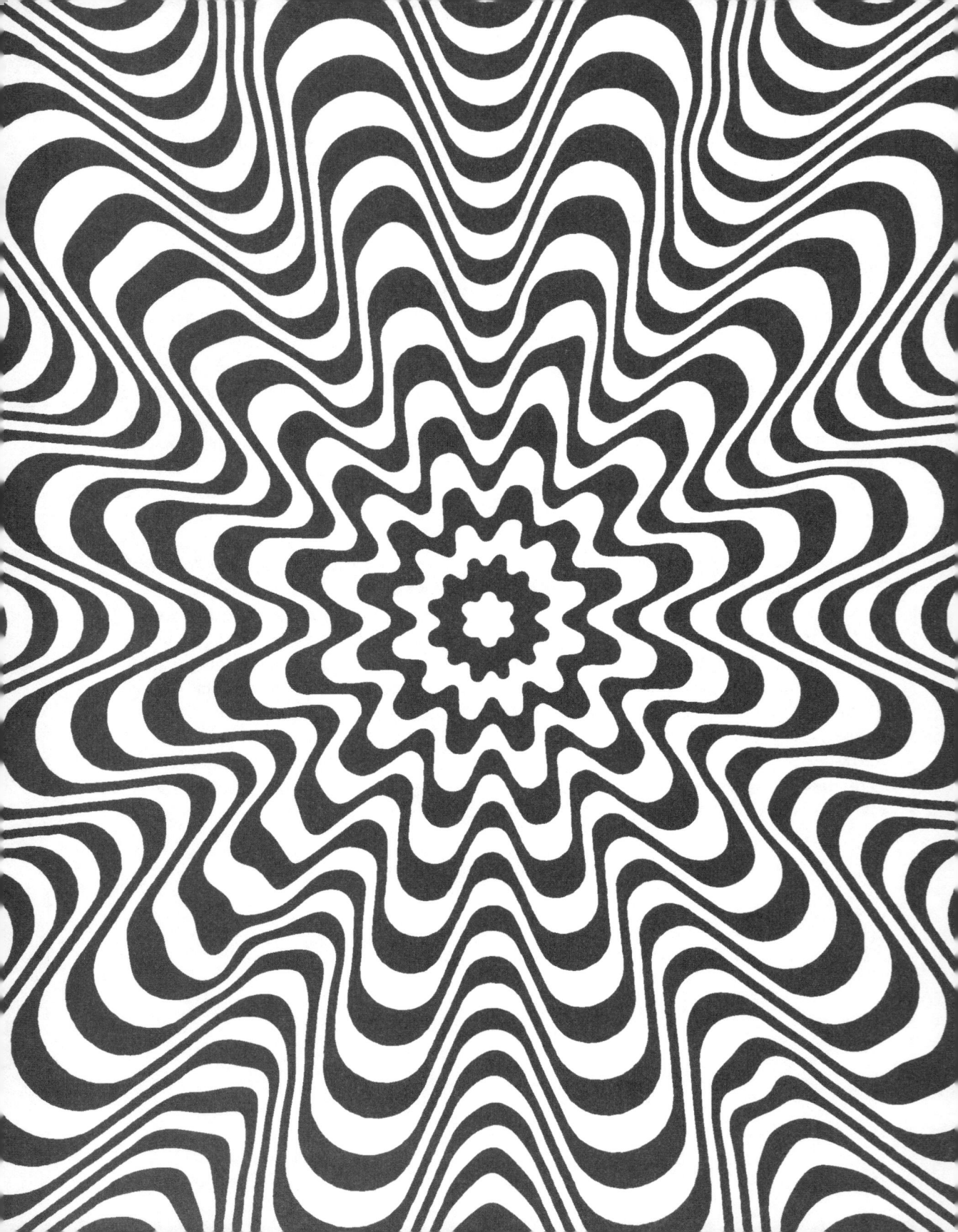

# CHAPTER 5

# MICRODOSING

------------------------------------------------------------------

Microdosing . . . it's not meant to do much, yet what does it do? Everything!

DR. ZACH WALSH, *clinical psychologist, lead researcher, Microdose.me*

Put simply, microdosing is the process of taking a sub-perceptual amount of a psychedelic (most commonly LSD or magic mushrooms, and more recently iboga root bark) on a regular basis in order to raise your mood, energy, and motivation; calm you down; or increase your patience with yourself and the world around you. *Sub-perceptual* means you do not feel any effect—no distortions of your visual field, no dazzling colors or oceanic feelings of unity with animals, clouds, or trees. At its best, the overall effects are said to be like a double espresso that lasts all day without the jitters. At its worst, you'll feel nothing.

It may take a little time and a few tweaks at the beginning of a microdosing routine to establish the right dose. From four years of personal experience microdosing with LSD, I learned that if the screen I've been staring at begins to go wavy, I was taking too much. If I felt a strange itchiness in my brain, if my heart was revving at a speed that was making concentration difficult, if all those unanswered emails were making me want to hurl my laptop across the room, I was taking too much. The good news is that these effects won't last long, and you can reduce your next dose.

Microdosing may be therapeutic, but it is definitely not psychedelic. The benefits should be subtle yet persistent.

When asked how microdosing benefits me, I can only say that it has a broad spectrum of subtle effects. It helps me feel better—about almost everything! It's not a happy pill; it works more quietly, as if addressing the underlying conditions that contribute to happiness. Some days my outlook is sunny in ways that surprise even me. It bumps up my motivation and makes me eager to get to work in the morning. Like aspirin, it doesn't call attention to itself. It's not dramatic. Wait! Let me rephrase that. The results of microdosing are dramatic—you just don't know they're happening until one day you wake up and you feel pretty damn good . . . or think, *Wow, that was a rough day, why am I still smiling?*

That said, psychedelics should not be thought of as just another supplement that will increase positive feelings of joy, happiness, or motivation. Although I've just extoled the virtues of microdosing, I have also learned that the truth is more complex: Even sub-perceptual doses of psychedelics cause you to feel more of everything, including the more painful emotions that we tend to run away from: sadness, fear, and anxiety. If you're not prepared to grapple with an expanded spectrum of emotion, microdosing may not be for you.

In her seminal book *A Really Good Day*, the charmingly irritable psychedelic skeptic Ayalet Waldman began microdosing with LSD after years of battling an intractable depression. She had tried SSRIs, mood stabilizers, and a pharmacopeia of other medications to no avail, so microdosing was a last resort. Her first day felt like nothing was happening, but once she was at work, she noticed the beauty of a tree through her window. Until that moment she had been incapable of appreciating beauty, and it struck her how rarely she felt "happy." After a few weeks of microdosing, her sadness lifted, her marital struggles eased, and her anxiety lowered, all of which unexpectedly fired up her creative output. "I became so immersed in my work that I didn't notice time passing," she recounts. "Getting lost in work, what's known as 'flow,' is one of the most exciting things about the process of creating . . . "[1]

Flow is the state of "intense emotional involvement and timelessness that comes from immersion in challenging activities," she continues. "It can happen when you are creating computer code or scaling a mountain. It's a gift that arrives rarely, when you are most focused and present." She wrote the first draft of her book in a month. Is there anyone who doesn't want more of that?

Before you rush headlong into a microdosing journey, let's be clear: There is scant clinical data about microdosing that support claims about its benefits. It first came to light in the 1960s and 1970s in the large underground LSD labs that were turning out millions of illegal doses. Despite their protective garments, the chemists working in those labs were constantly exposed to sub-threshold doses—it was impossible to keep flocculent particles from dissolving in the aqueous tissue of the eye, for example. As the orange groves in what is now Silicon Valley were replaced by Intel offices, programmers who were staying up for days on end also found their way to microdosing. Some claimed it sparked insights that today power some of our most ubiquitous technologies.

Now, as it was then, microdosing remains difficult to study. Very few granting foundations will support a proposal that gives subjects illegal substances they self-administer at home. Most small clinical studies conclude that microdosing does little to nothing, while self-reported studies describe benefits ranging from enhanced creativity, focus, and empathy to improvements in a range of mental health conditions.

It's not surprising that the results of self-reported studies are more positive. People who have better outcomes are more likely to join studies or post on Reddit than people who feel nothing. The latter group tends to avoid studies, which is one of the main problems with the reliability of self-reporting.

The other challenge with self-reporting is what researchers call expectancy effects. People who take a supplement to boost energy will likely feel more energetic. "That doesn't mean it's a false effect," says Dr. Zach Walsh, a clinical psychologist and professor at University of British Columbia. "Something inert can still have an effect. But microdosing isn't inert. LSD or psilocybin cross the blood brain barrier and antagonize serotonin receptors.

It's possible that these neurochemical effects interact with expectancies, so it needn't be either or. Expectancies are an important aspect of many well-validated drug effects.

"I'm a big fan of small changes and little effects accumulating over time," he continues. "If microdosing has a modest positive effect on your relationships, if it helps you to go to sleep easier, if you drink one less beer a day, all of those subtle things could have a broad effect on general health."

If nothing else, he adds, it shouldn't be illegal. "It's one of those things where the benefits may be modest, but the risks are modest as well, in which case, leave people alone."

## Risks and Adverse Effects

"There's very rarely a biological free lunch," author, podcaster, and psychedelic entrepreneur Tim Ferriss tweeted in 2019. "LSD and other psychedelics are serotonin receptor agonists—they activate serotonin like SSRIs, but in a different mechanism." Ferriss's concern was that even low doses may impact the brain's serotonin production in unknown ways and throw endogenous production out of whack.

Other psychopharmacologists argue that whatever the long-term risks may be, they'll be fewer than those associated with prescribed antidepressants. "I think when people get around to researching microdosing, it's going to demonstrate positive effects that are better than conventional antidepressants, which are awful," said David Presti, professor of neurobiology in the Department of Molecular and Cell Biology at the University of California–Berkeley. "SSRIs have all kinds of side effects and we have no idea, really, what they're doing.

They cost a lot of money and are marketed with all kinds of flimflam."[2]

However, some people may be more prone to the mild adverse effects of microdosing. It can increase anxious feelings, so it's not recommended for people diagnosed with generalized anxiety disorder. Those people can try lowering the dose or switching the drug, but if feelings of anxiety persist, microdosing is probably not a solution for them.

People who have red-green color blindness should also proceed cautiously, as they are more susceptible to developing tracers as a side effect.

## Clinical Evidence

Two of the largest mushroom microdosing studies were both published in *Nature* in 2022—but they reached contradictory conclusions. The first, a double-blind, placebo-controlled study with thirty-four participants, found no evidence "to support enhanced well-being, creativity, and cognitive function."[3] The second self-reported study followed 953 microdosers and 180 non-microdosing controls for a month and found "small- to medium-sized improvements in mood and mental health that were consistent across gender and age."[4]

These two studies are a microcosm of the literature as a whole, with different experimental methods reaching different conclusions. Despite these divergent results and approaches, both studies were considered strong enough to be published in one of the world's top science journals within months of each other.

While there is no scientific consensus, there is mounting evidence that microdosing *may* help people with conditions including chronic pain and ADHD along with the usual suspects: depression, anxiety, PTSD.

## PAIN REDUCTION

One study gave single doses of 5, 10, and 20 mcg of LSD or a placebo to twenty-four volunteers over several days.[5] Researchers then assessed their pain tolerance by asking them to submerge their hands in a tank of cold water for as long as they could endure. The 20 mcg dose of LSD reduced pain perception by 20 percent. The analgesic effects of the LSD were equally strong an hour and a half and five hours after administration. Researchers compared analgesic effects of microdosing LSD to those of opioids.

## ADHD: MICRODOSING VERSUS ADDERALL*

A recent two-part study from the Netherlands examined microdosing among adults with ADHD.[6] Part one found improvements in emotional regulation and empathy in participants who microdosed on their own, regardless of concurrent ADHD medication use. Part two compared microdosing with conventional ADHD meds: One group microdosed, and the other continued treatment as usual with their standard medication.

After four weeks, the microdosers had less severe ADHD symptoms compared with the treatment-as-usual group. While these results are promising, it is worth noting that neither part of the study was placebo-controlled, and participants were free to use whatever substance they wanted (though over 90 percent used psilocybin mushrooms).

## Crowdsourced Evidence

The difficulty of studying microdosing in lab settings has led James Fadiman and Paul Stamets to independently gather reports over the years from thousands of "citizen scientists" to paint a cohesive picture of self-reported evidence.

## LSD MICRODOSING: THE FADIMAN 3-DAY PROTOCOL

James Fadiman is a Harvard- and Stanford-trained author, researcher, philosopher, and dedicated psychedelic OG who no longer uses psychedelics. He was the more straitlaced collaborator of Timothy Leary and Richard Alpert in the 1960s. He has been investigating these substances on and off, but mostly on, since 1962. To Fadiman, the 230,000 Reddit contributors who openly share their microdosing results are not to be discounted: "They tell you more than twelve people in a Johns Hopkins study," he has said.[7]

Fadiman has surveyed thousands of LSD microdosers about their experiences. Most were taking 10 to 15 mcg on day one, which they identified as their most "on" day. On day two, people generally reported sunnier moods than day one. On day three, they felt almost nothing, which Fadiman theorizes is a "reset day" in which psychedelic residue clears the synapses and reduces chances of developing tolerance. Based on these findings, Fadiman came up with a sixty-day protocol followed by a week off to clear the receptors. He never intended it to become an "official" regimen, but it is known today as "the Fadiman 3-Day Protocol." (See next page.)

Among the more surprising outcomes were the unexpected benefits realized by some microdosers. One of Fadiman's subjects began microdosing to elevate his mood, but he was

---

* Terence McKenna reported that Albert Hofmann "believed that Sandoz could have brought to market a small dose version of LSD that could have competed with Ritalin or Adderall."

## BENEFITS OF MICRODOSING, ACCORDING TO MICRODOSE.ME

- Enhanced mindfulness, specifically the ability to connect with the present moment rather than being stuck in the past or the future
- Reduced anxiety and depression
- Improved mood, memory, and cognition
- Enhanced creative thinking
- Improved motor skills
- Improved hearing and vision
- A greater sense of interconnection
- Relief from PTSD (post-traumatic stress disorder) symptoms
- Reduced incidence of neuropathy

able to quit smoking after a five-year, pack-a-day habit. Another broke a weed habit without trying to. A stutterer stopped stuttering.

Students reported that microdosing is a good substitute for Adderall. Migraine sufferers noted a 70 to 90 percent reduction in the occurrence of headaches. A few were happily surprised to find relief from cluster headaches (though it's generally agreed that high-dose treatment with LSD or psilocybin is more effective).

### MUSHROOM MICRODOSING: THE STAMETS STACK

The medicinal mushroom evangelist Paul Stamets devised another protocol called the Stamets Stack, which blends psilocybin mushroom and lion's mane mycelium with niacin to speed the compounds into the bloodstream. To investigate efficacy, he cocreated the Microdose.me app, which collects data from twenty-four

thousand users on cognitive performance and mental health. Users reported statistically significant reductions in depression and trauma, along with improvements in mood. A small number of participants are also showing promising results on a new app-based motor skills test; the greatest improvements were seen in people over fifty-five—surprising, given that motor skills usually decline with age.

The "tap test" is not about how you feel. It's a physiological gauge that involves tapping your finger as quickly as you can on a screen to measure cognitive control over motor skills. Tapping a screen sounds like a sad little measure of success, but, as Stamets explained to a standing-room presentation at the 2023 MAPS Psychedelic Science conference, "It takes an enormously complex set of neurons . . . over six regions of the brain to accomplish this . . . It's playing piano, playing a trombone. *It's walking into the bathroom at 80 years old and not falling down!*" [Emphasis mine.]

Zach Walsh, Stamets's academic and far more measured Microdose.me collaborator, agrees that early results on the tap test, if not groundbreaking, are promising. The sample size of fifty is small, so Walsh is waiting to replicate results before making any big pronouncements. But if the results prove out, Walsh says he'll be "blown away. Slow tapping is a solid index of psychomotor ability, which is an early indicator of cognitive decline, Parkinson's disease, and Alzheimer's. It's not a diagnosis, but it's not irrelevant. It's somewhere between. It's a marker."

## Two Microdosing Protocols
### THE FADIMAN 3-DAY LSD PROTOCOL
- Confirm the strength of your LSD. In the

US, a typical tab of LSD is said to be 100 micrograms, but this can vary.*

- Dilute one tab of LSD or 100 mcg liquid LSD in ten tablespoons of distilled water. Do not use tap water, as it often contains chlorine, which kills LSD.
- Shake well before each use—LSD falls out of solution and drops to the bottom of the bottle.
- Take 1 to 1.5 tablespoons every three days. Be sure to set your calendar as a reminder.
- Every sixty days, stop for one week to "resensitize" your receptors. The pause is unresearched but generally agreed upon by the global community of microdosers.

*Note:* It's a good idea to begin on a day when you don't have to work or have much to do, just in case. If you are feeling uncomfortable or experiencing any signs of being high, you are taking too much. Reduce your next dose and continue until you find your sweet spot.

## THE STAMETS STACK

Stacking is the process of combining psilocybin, niacin (vitamin $B_3$), and medicinal lion's mane mushrooms to get synergistic potency. Psilocybin[8] and lion's mane[9] have been shown to create new neuronal connections and repair existing neurological damage. Niacin acts as a vasodilator and helps to speed psilocin across the blood-brain barrier and throughout the nervous system.

### Psilocybin

In addition to everything you've already read about psilocybin, Stamets believes it can make

---

# MICRODOSING MISAPPREHENSIONS

**"I'm not feeling anything specific, so nothing is happening."** Microdosing appears to exert a more holistic effect on the body and manifests in ways that are difficult to pin down or label. Effects include higher energy, sharper decision-making, and increased motivation and focus. Remember, aspirin or CBD effectively reduce pain in quiet ways that often go unnoticed.

**Microdosing is often referred to as "tripping light,"** but it's totally different from tripping. There is no shift in normal waking consciousness. It can, however, cause significant shifts in physical ailments, but the shifts occur subtly and can take time to be felt. Some migraine sufferers report reduced occurrences from four per month to one every two months. Menstrual cramps are also reported to be less severe.

**"My intention always drives the outcome."** People start microdosing for one effect, but then they notice: *My shingles went away . . . the symptoms of my Lyme disease have eased up . . . I have fewer headaches.* Thousands of microdosers have reported changes that had nothing to do with the reason they started.

---

you smarter, kinder, and more courageous, which, unsurprisingly, is why his MAPS lecture

---

* Learn how the new-to-market QTest assesses potency in chapter 7, "Harm Reduction."

was titled "How Psilocybin Mushrooms Can Help Save the World." Regardless, small doses are said to stimulate neurogenesis and do not interfere with functioning.

### Niacin

Niacin is naturally present in many foods like beef liver and brown rice and is a common dietary supplement. According to a 2019 review,[10] optimal intake may delay neurodegeneration, but more research is needed to support this claim. Since niacin acts as a flushing agent and causes vasodilation, a low dose is thought to distribute healing molecules into the extremities where much neuronal development occurs.

### Lion's Mane

Lion's mane (*Hericium erinaceus*) is a non-psychedelic mushroom known to positively affect brain health and reduce inflammation. It has been used in traditional Chinese medicine to treat neurasthenia (chronic fatigue). Two of its constituents, erinacines and hericenones, contain neurogenerative[11] and neuroprotective[12] properties—at least that's what animal studies show.

### Preparing Your Mushroom Microdose

- Grind mushrooms in a coffee grinder. Allow the grinds to sit in the grinder for an hour to avoid spreading magic mushroom dust across your kitchen counter. You could also enclose the entire device in a large freezer bag before removing the lid.
- Weigh ingredients on an inexpensive electronic kitchen scale. Scales accurate to 0.1 to 1.0 grams cost about $20.
- Gently place in gelcaps.

Stamets's stacking formula for a 154-pound (70 kg) individual is:

- 0.5–1 mg *Psilocybe cubensis*
- 100–500 mg lion's mane mushrooms
- 25–50 mg niacin (vitamin $B_3$)*

### The Stamets Stack Protocol

- Days 1–4: stacking days (take one dose per day)
- Days 5–7: take a break (do not dose)
- Days 8–11: stacking days
- Days 12–14: break days

Continue this cycle for four to six weeks, followed by a reset period (no dosing) of two to four weeks.

### How Safe Is the Stack?

This is yet to be determined, but since the individual components of the stack are recognized as safe at higher doses and do not incur long-term adverse effects, we can assume the same for sub-perceptual doses.

The Amsterdam-based Microdosing Institute, which has coached over five thousand people, deems the stack inexpensive and safe. If you're interested in working with a microdosing coach, the institute's coaches are all volunteers so the price is very right.

---

* Taking too much niacin can cause an allergic reaction. It can also interact with alcohol and other drugs such as diabetes medications. It is not recommended for people with liver or kidney disease, diabetes, gout, or peptic ulcer disease.

There are few studies about niacin in pregnant women, lactating mothers, seniors, or children.

Common side effects of 50 mg or more of niacin include sensations of tingling, burning, itching, and skin flushing. These symptoms are not toxic and disappear after thirty minutes.

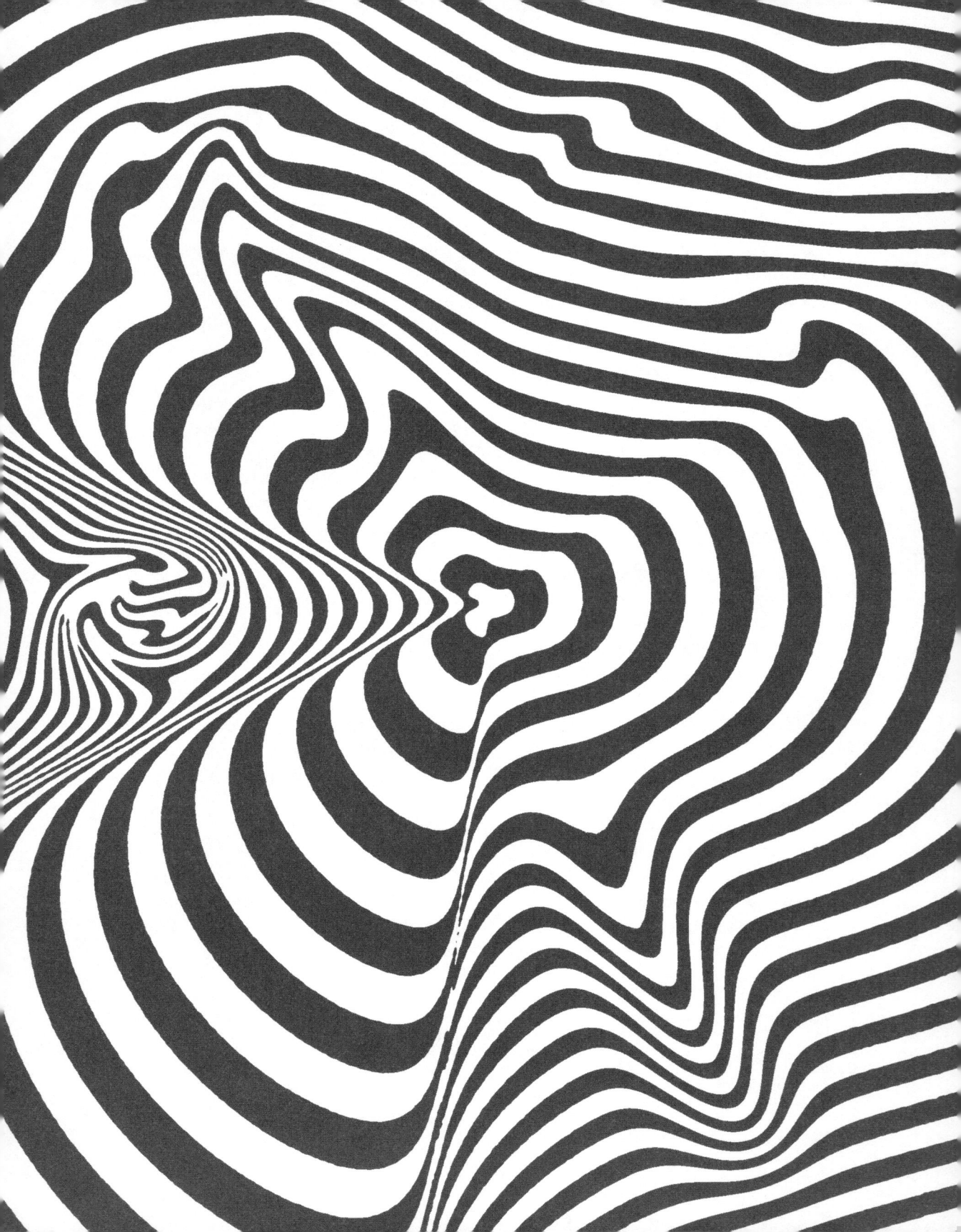

# CHAPTER 6

# COUPLES AND PSYCHEDELICS

E ver since therapists in the 1970s proclaimed that six hours of therapy on MDMA was the equivalent of a year's worth of therapy, it has become a widely repeated (and little researched) refrain. In fact couples use MDMA, psilocybin, ketamine, LSD, and 2C-B in many ways that aren't necessarily therapeutic: to find more warmth, forgiveness, and equanimity; to add spark to their sex lives; to build new bridges to intimacy; and to call it quits without losing sight of each other's humanity. And this isn't exclusive to romantic couples. Friends, and what psychologist Eli Finkle terms our *"other* significant others"—nontraditional long-term platonic commitments—are using psychedelics to explore the liminal spaces that exist between one person's consciousness and another's.

Research on psychedelics and relationships has been scant, but the few studies that have been conducted generally report positive outcomes. One of the most widely cited is a 1986 paper by Dr. George R. Greer and Requa Tolbert, who studied the effects of MDMA on twenty-nine couples.[1]

Unsurprisingly, most couples were able to communicate with much less fear, but each individual also reported positive mood changes, tighter focus on life goals, and increased spiritual dimensionality.* Only two couples reported negative changes in their relationship. Among Greer and Tolbert's conclusions: "The single best use of MDMA is to facilitate more direct communication between people involved in a significant emotional relationship. Not only is communication enhanced during the session, but afterward . . . . This ability can not only help resolve existing conflicts, but it can also prevent future ones from occurring due to unexpressed fears or misunderstandings."

## MDMA FOR RELATIONSHIP REINVIGORATION

Ayalet Waldman, author of *A Really Good Day*, doesn't use drugs, not even weed. Occasionally she'll use CBD, but that's the extent of her experimentation. Sasha Shulgin and his wife, Ann, whom Ayalet knew through teaching at UC Berkeley, convinced Ayalet and her husband, the author Michael Chabon, to try MDMA as a tool for relationship reinvigoration. Their marriage was not in distress, but she

*CONTINUED*

---

* In more recent studies, MDMA has been found to encourage easier expression of emotions; reduced pain at being criticized or rejected; increased ability to identify emotions in others; decreased defensiveness; and increased ability to stay in the present moment.

and Michael have four kids and several jobs each, so a buildup of tension is inevitable. "The PTSD of a long marriage," is how she puts it.

The couple used MDMA to "spend six hours talking about everything that has come up for us from a place of absolute love and commitment. MDMA allows us to talk about our issues, but from a place of connection and love," Waldman has said. "That one experience sustains us for as long as two years. It's really remarkable."[2]

These findings are being echoed today. Dr. Bessel van der Kolk is the author of *The Body Keeps the Score*, founder of the Trauma Research Foundation, and a lead researcher in Phase III studies on MDMA-assisted therapy for PTSD. He has been consistently impressed by the way MDMA enables couples in distress to surface difficult, seemingly unspeakable truths.

One thing that really struck me in the secondary analysis [of the trials] was the alexithymia scales. Alexithymia is a very big word that means "inability to identify what you're feeling."

What you see in the MDMA-assisted therapy is that people are able to say, "This is who I am. This is what I feel. This is what's important and unimportant to me, and I'm no longer dependent on you for dictating what I feel."

We had couples in very nasty, abusive relationships. And rather than saying, "My husband is such a terrible person who does all these terrible things to me," they were able to reframe their thinking: "I'm actually married to a very dysfunctional person. I need to negotiate what I need in a calm way because that's what I need."

I was astounded that two of our subjects were able to negotiate exiting their relationships in a calm and mindful way without blowing up or becoming threatening.

That is really stunning, their sense of themselves coming online.[3]

Van der Kolk warns that MDMA can also open a Pandora's box of emotion, and he advises couples on the edge to use it only in a supported environment. His idea for lowering the costs of MDMA-assisted couples counseling is to create a program that trains laypeople to facilitate couples work in exchange for treatment. "The trauma field started with laypeople from the feminist movement in Cambridge, Massachusetts, and peer support groups for veterans. Both groups did much better with peers than with professionals," he says.

That's a lovely idea, but couples aren't waiting for a program like this to begin. Instead, they're using MDMA and other psychedelics on their own to explore the dynamics of their duo.

## How Couples Are Using Psychedelics

Dr. Ido Cohen is a clinical psychologist in the San Francisco Bay Area who trains psychedelic-assisted therapists and runs his own integration circles. In 2023, he and fellow therapist and facilitator Deanna Rogers conducted a small retrospective study (unpublished as of this writing) with fifteen couples (straight, gay, otherwise; some with kids, some without) to learn how psychedelics can help people explore their partnerships. "We saw that couples are doing beautiful things on their own but there were also some surprising gaps," Cohen says. The insights gathered from this small sample jibe with those of other therapists I've interviewed, and are worthy of discussion.

## WHAT THEY'RE USING

Most couples journeying together turn to MDMA or ketamine. Lower-dose psilocybin and LSD come in second place. DMT, ayahuasca, and full-dose ibogaine are too inward-acting for relational joint experiences.

Says Cohen: "MDMA can be good for people who want something more gentle. If they have difficulty or fear staying in relationships, MDMA can help them be more connected. It's useful for people struggling with intimacy and it can provide a more cohesive experience. Ketamine has a similar action—it decreases nervous system activation so people are more present and less reactive." Most couples used a low-dose therapeutic lozenge that lasts for two or three hours.*

Psilocybin and LSD can bring on laughter and engender feelings of oneness and well-being, but high doses can send each partner on their own trip for some part of the journey. Visuals can get intense, and thoughts can blitz through the mind faster than words come out of the mouth, especially with acid. But both substances can catalyze connection because they tear down your walls and mute your filters. This can have the aftereffect of "changing the way [couples] think about the relationship," says Cohen.

## HOW THEY PREPARE

Most couples spend time creating a space to trip apart from their everyday living arrangements. Some set up a tent in the backyard or close off and decorate a specific room of the house.

## NAMING THE THING

Dr. Erica Zelfand treated a couple that had been together for forty years in an MDMA-supported session. Despite four decades together, this man and woman were not a great match and they knew it. Their adult children didn't want their parents to do the session fearing it would end in divorce.

MDMA enabled the couple to "name the thing," says Zelfand. "They said, 'We got together when we were young for unhealthy reasons, but we have so much water under the bridge and we are loyal, so let's not break our forty year bond.' And they ended up choosing to stay together.

"In our culture, we measure the success of a relationship by how long it lasts, and that includes how long people can endure their mutual suffering. That's not a measure of success even if it lasts for sixty years. I've seen MDMA help couples define what success looks like and then align with what that means. And sometimes it means 'Thank you so much, and I'm setting you free now.'"

---

* A few couples noted that too frequent use can lead to cravings.

Others repair to a safe place in the forest or near the sea, away from any possible interruptions.

While they expend effort on setting, only a third of the couples engage in conscious preparation; those who did set intentions didn't look far below the surface. "We were surprised that so few couples seemed to understand that creating a nuanced intention is actually the beginning of the journey," Cohen says.

Many couples said they were hoping to "work" on their connection, but as Cohen points out, "connection" has many shades of meaning. *Do you want to be able to talk more vulnerably with me? Why can't you do that? Are we talking enough about sex or are we avoiding the elephant in the room?*

His advice? Plumb deeper to bring important topics to the forefront of consciousness. "With a deeper distillation couples might get to, *'My hope is that we can use the psychedelic to talk about why I feel scared to share certain vulnerable things,'* or *'What happens if I get so turned on that I become lustful but you don't want to be touched?'*"

Talking beforehand is so important, especially regarding consent about sex, or pressuring each other to talk or be together during the trip, or doing something that isn't agreed upon in advance. If couples can uncover the blocks, hopes, and desires before they journey, it can open more than "Let's work on our connection."

Another gap in preparation seemed to be that only 15 percent talked about dosing. "The general approach was 'Let's each take what we want,'" says Cohen. "Individuals were aware of their own sensitivities, like 'I need X milligrams or X micrograms to feel something,' but they weren't aware of what they needed to be on the same consciousness frequency."

## ADDING SIZZLE TO SEX

Over half of the couples viewed psychedelics as a way to fire up their erotic lives. Cohen defines *eros* as the measure of aliveness that exists between two people and notes that erotic charges can come from many directions.

"Talking intimately, making out, full on penetrative sex, all are aspects of eros," he says. "Under the psychedelic some couples realized they don't have as much play as they once did. And when there's no play, there's less foreplay and less foreplay means less arousal and less exciting sex."

For others, the simple act of touching, or even talking about touching, was an invitation to deeper connection. (See "The Three-Minute Game," page 161.)

Three couples described having what Cohen defined as "spiritual or transpersonal sex," the experience of having their energies merge as if they were having sex in a different dimension—something akin to what Sara, a twenty-eight-year old marketing executive, told Vice.com in a 2022 article called "Love and Other Drugs: The Couples Using Psychedelics as a Way to Get Closer." "Acid strips your feelings down to the core, allowing you to feel everything on the deepest level. When you have the face of the love of your life in your hands, that deep sense of belonging and connection is simply unmatched. We've seen our souls intertwine and felt strands of energy tie us together. You simply don't get that alone or with friends."[4]

## FULL ALLOWANCE

Two-thirds of the couples said their journeys were more satisfying if their partners encouraged them to have every emotion without judgment. "If they're touching each other and suddenly one starts to sob or laugh uncontrollably, the other doesn't try to stop it. They allow it to happen without trying to fix it," says Cohen.

"If some big emotion or trauma arises, it's better to lead with curiosity, *'Do you want to tell me more?'* or *'Do you need to be in your own space?'* Three-quarters of the couples said honest disclosure combined with their partner's full acceptance was crucial to successfully tripping together."

## FANTASIES

Psychedelics are an invitation into the unconscious, so it's no surprise that sharing fantasies of all sorts was a common occurrence. Some were sexual in nature but others included big-picture desires about how the couple could move forward. Psychedelics made it safer to surface the long-term desires that can go unspoken in the bustle of everyday life. With parents, this often involved discussions of different approaches to raising their kids.

## INTIMACY AND SENSUALITY

Almost three-quarters of the couples engaged in sensory practices. Some explored nonsexual touch. Others simply stared into each other's eyes, which, Cohen says, "seems to invite an intense working through of psychological projections with less fear and more forgiveness. *'I see you getting older,'* or *'I can see your pain,'* were common observations. Another said, *'I saw all the things you had to go through to get to me and I felt so much more compassion because your life was rough.'* Notably, all the couples landed in a place where they felt the essence of their partner and a deep love for the human being beneath all of those layers."

## INTEGRATION

Surprisingly to Cohen and Rogers, only a quarter of these couples integrated with their partners; most spoke to a friend or therapist or joined an integration circle. Only 50 percent journaled following their experience.

Not integrating can lead to disappointment down the line, says Cohen. "Some people get really excited in the 'sparkle period' following the journey, but after a week or two it's gone and depression can set in or they can form a narrative of disappointment, *'I thought it was meaningful, but it was an illusion'*—which contradicts the life-changing revelations you had a week ago.

"We see a big hole in the integration process because there isn't a structure that helps couples continue exploring after the journey ends," Cohen continues. "Integration should be about opening, not closing. It should give you more questions about how to keep the conversation going."

## TIGHTER, LIGHTER, FAIRER FIGHTERS

Overall, 60 percent of Cohen and Rogers's couples said their psychedelic journeys left them more attuned to themselves and their partners. Forty percent got insight into their own trauma and how it plays out in partnership.

Eighty-five percent said it deepened their intimacy, increased their openness and willingness to forgive, and lowered their reactivity and defensiveness. Importantly, it changed the way they fight. "When you see the preciousness and the beautiful spirit that's in your partner, it's more difficult to be malicious," says Cohen.

Dr. Zelfand has seen a similar pattern in the couples she's worked with: "In my experience,

## WHEN PSYCHEDELICS COME BETWEEN YOU AND YOUR PARTNER

"Psychedelics can be divisive if both partners aren't participating," says Dr. Erica Zelfand. "This issue isn't often discussed, but the psychedelic can actually start to feel like the other woman or man."

This most commonly occurs when one person goes on a retreat and the other stays home. The retreatant makes new friends and has a powerful experience, leaving the spouse back home feeling overlooked or threatened. It has happened frequently enough that Zelfand has prepared an information packet for the at-home partner (righttoheal.com/friend-family-retreat-preparation). "It explains the experience your partner is about to have and that they may be different when they come home—and that can be a good thing."

Another source of division occurs when one part of the couple is pretending to support the other partner's psychedelicizing, but in fact resents it. "That can feel like a polyamory dynamic and can explode," says Zelfand. "But when both partners are on board, it can be a beautiful, powerful relationship saving tool—unrivaled in its efficacy in my observation."

couples tend to fight about the same thing over and over. Even the happiest couple has different iterations of the same fight on the same topic repeatedly. MDMA slows things down so you can see where you normally get hooked so you're able to hear what your partner has been trying to get you to hear for five or ten years without going on defense. Even if you don't agree with what they're saying, it allows you to hear it and empathize, *'This is how it must feel for them.'"*

### Psychedelics and Sexual Arousal

Psychedelics may work as aphrodisiacs, but they are not sexual panaceas. They can expand and explore sexuality, but their greatest use seems to be deepening the emotional connections that lead to deeper sex. "The relaxation and disinhibition effect of many psychedelics is what most people respond to," Ann Shulgin noted in a 2002 interview with MAPS.[5] "If you're in a sexual situation what

> **"Mushrooms can facilitate a great, giddy laugh, an underappreciated erotic enhancement."**

you want is to drop the tension and the over-activity of the intellect. And most psychedelics do that."

## LSD AND SEX

"LSD is the most powerful aphrodisiac ever discovered by man," so said Timothy Leary, a master of the grandiose pronouncement. But to this, the best response is, "Well, maybe." Lots of couples say they've had ecstatic, multidimensional, otherworldly sex on LSD, but it's not known to be a heart connector. What happens depends on the dose, the environment, and, of course, the person you're with.

## MDMA AND SEX

While MDMA can increase certain forms of arousal for women—several studies report enhanced vaginal lubrication and desire, and satisfaction ratings were through the roof[6]—almost half (40 percent) of men report not being able to have an erection or ejaculation on Ecstasy. If you're a man planning a wild night on MDMA, know that sex often happens after the effects have worn off, and often not until the following day.

It's considered safe for healthy men to use Cialis or Viagra with pure MDMA to induce erections, but when MDMA is really hitting, erections can seem beside the point.

## 2C-B AND SEX

MDMA gets all of the love-drug glory, but the lesser known 2C-B was chemist Sasha Shulgin's favorite drug for sex. "If there is anything ever found to be an effective aphrodisiac, it will probably be patterned after 2C-B in structure," he wrote in *PiHKAL*. Several therapists of the

1970s and 1980s reported it pairing well with MDMA.* Those who don't experience 2C-B as insistently sexual seem to appreciate the fact that it doesn't get in the way.

- Compared with MDMA, 2C-B is shorter acting—it lasts about three to four hours compared with four to six.
- It's also less stimulating and not as speedy as MDMA. It's more a mescaline derivative and belongs to an adjacent class of psychedelics, phenethylamines. Instead of being hyperstimulated, people describe feeling grounded in the body.
- Raised hairs, muscle spasms, erections and other signs of physical arousal can occur throughout a 2C-B trip.

## MAGIC MUSHROOMS AND SEX

Magic mushrooms typically don't spark sexual arousal or intimacy as directly as MDMA or 2C-B. But psilocybin can boost empathy and interconnection, which can ease sexual challenges or anxiety. It can also facilitate a great, giddy laugh, and laughter is an underappreciated erotic enhancement.

Psilocybin does combine nicely with kanna. One 1929 report said of kanna users: "Their animal spirits became animated, their eyes sparkled, and their faces were marked by laughter and happiness. A thousand charming ideas arose in them, a gentle joy that amused itself over the simplest of jests." Hot!

## LOW-DOSE KETAMINE AND SEX

It seems baffling that a dissociative anesthetic can produce sexual sensations, but plenty of

---

* Typically, 2C-B was administered two hours after MDMA.

people find the euphoric, floaty effects of ketamine sexually lubricating.

### Advantages to K-Sex

- Users report relaxed muscles and reduced anxiety.
- For those who are into kink or who like rougher play, it is a way to find more pleasure within the context of pain.
- Increased libido or heightened sensuality are reported.
- A sensation of two bodies dissolving into one can be brought on by the somatic dissociative effects of K, leading to a more potent bonding.
- There's no hangover with ketamine.
- Used under supervision, it can help heal sexual traumas, which can, in turn, raise libido.

### Limitations to K-Sex

- Too high a dose can disconnect you from your body.
- If men overindulge, they may not get hard.
- It can lower inhibitions, leading to unsafe or nonconsensual sex.
- Repeated use can lead to tolerance and addiction, so use it mindfully and occasionally.
- Warning: Do not mix ketamine with GHB, alcohol, or any suppressants. The combination can be dangerous to the respiratory system.

## THE DOWNSIDES OF PSYCHEDELICS AND SEX

Now that you've heard about some of the rapturous libidinous possibilities, be aware that psychedelics can also ruin sexual encounters, especially at high doses and in uncomfortable environments.

## WHY DON'T WE KNOW MORE ABOUT PSYCHEDELIC SEX?

Our understanding of the relationship between sex and drugs remains extremely limited. Researchers have a tendency to focus on associations between drug use and "risky" sexual behavior, such as how multiple sexual partners can increase your chances of contracting an STI. Studies also tend to highlight the links between drug use and "impaired" sexual function, such as erectile dysfunction or difficulties achieving an orgasm.[7] This creates an "official" picture of sex and drugs that is disproportionately focused on the negatives.

And on erections.

Science knows little about women's experiences of sex on psychedelics and what female enhancement might feel like in these contexts. Since the FDA approval of Viagra for treating erectile dysfunction in the 1990s, there have been calls for the development of a female counterpart. But the medical condition that such a drug might "treat" is unclear.[8]

At high doses, you might prefer staring at your favorite painting for hours, diving into your own subconscious, or exploring the ramifications of existentialism rather than the curve of your partner's back. You may need to leave the room to be alone for a while. Indifference is rarely a sexual turn-on. To preclude this, well

# WHY ARE POLICYMAKERS SO AFRAID OF PLEASURE?

Being better informed about pleasure could benefit society as a whole, not just those who use drugs. The US government spends significant time and money trying to prevent drug-related harm. Many activities carry a risk, such as driving a car, but we don't try to reduce traffic fatalities by banning driving. Instead, we educate drivers to minimize the risks of getting behind the wheel.

When it comes to drugs, policymakers still believe that prohibition and scare tactics work. But adults across demographic categories use drugs, so they deserve policies that are more mature than the current offerings of denial and ignorance. For a more detailed exploration of this topic, have a look at Dr. Carl Hart's provocative and refreshingly honest book, *Drug Use for Grown-Ups*.

in advance of your journey, grant your partner the freedom to be alone or withdrawn for as long as they may need to be.

It goes without saying, but chemicals alone do not nurture sexual desire. The bedrocks of desire are trust, connection, emotional stability, and self-confidence. So, rather than focusing on psychedelics to fix a sexual issue, first consider your mental and emotional barriers to passion.

## THE THREE-MINUTE GAME*

The Three-Minute Game was made famous by Betty Martin, a multimodal bodyworker. It's a simple but powerful exploration of power and surrender that can offer couples insights into intimacy and desire. Betty suggests trying it first clothed and in a nonsexual context. I think that's a good idea before experimenting with it on psychedelics.

It consists of each partner asking the other two questions. The first is:

1. How do you want me to touch you for three minutes?

    The answer should be something your partner can allow with a full heart. If there's any objection, talk about it.

    Set a timer for three minutes. Then reverse roles.

The second round begins with this question:

2. How do you want to touch me for three minutes?

    Many people have never been asked this question, says Martin, so it can sound confusing at first. *What do I want to do to my partner with my hands, feet, lips, toes, mouth?* Ask yourself if this is a gift you can give with a full heart.

    Set a timer for three minutes and then reverse roles.

---

* You don't have to be a couple to play this game. It is sensual but isn't necessarily sexual. It can be played clothed or naked, with psychedelics or without. When you're playing on a psychedelic, it's useful to write down the questions and refer to them frequently.

After four rounds, you may come away with the understanding that asking for what you want actually works!

## INTIMACY ENHANCEMENTS FOR MDMA PARTNERS[*]

### Altoid Invigoration

While tripping, sucking on and sharing mints can really boost both kissing and oral sex. Halls cough drops seem to be the strong preference for oral sex, as menthol can be extremely invigorating.

### Body Exploration

In this exercise, one person is an inactive participant and simply lies there or stands completely naked, allowing their partner to explore their body with their eyes, nose, hands, tongue . . . Partners can begin clothed and strip as things progress, or be naked from the outset. Blindfold optional.

There is no stress or pressure on the explorer to provide pleasure during this experience; they are simply enjoying their partner's body. You may be surprised at what you learn.

### Compliment Shower

Intimacy isn't just sex. The empathogenic qualities of MDMA amplify feelings. While sitting, standing, or even lying down, look your partner directly in the eyes and tell them everything you love about them, from their physical characteristics to the things they do, their personality traits, and your happiest memories with them. Watch their face as your words land.

### Cuddling

One of the greatest feelings in the world is simply cuddling on Ecstasy—it's soothing and thrilling at the same time. Hold each other close and find sincere comfort and warmth. Cuddle up under a blanket on the couch, by a warm fire, lying in bed, standing, fully clothed, completely naked . . . the choice is yours. Talk, listen to music, or stay silent, whatever feels right.

### Face Massage

A face massage is an absolute must. Besides the obvious manipulation of the face with massaging hands, try using the soft soles of the feet, or drag long hair across the face for a different sensation. Massage oil can be used for a new feeling as well, but be careful of eye irritants. Plain water is often enough; try experimenting with hot and cold.

### Feet and Toes

The feet and toes present remarkable erogenous zones with extraordinary sensitivity. They are also neglected areas when it comes to sex.

Users report time and time again that having their toes sucked (aka shrimping) is intensely enjoyable on Ecstasy. Do not neglect the webbing—the skin between the toes. One user described experiencing an orgasm just from having the skin between her toes licked. That should give you an idea of the potential.

The arches of the foot can be especially sensitive, and you can scrunch your feet to create ridges or wrinkles on the soles, resulting in different textures and sensations.

Also, try separating your partner's toes with your fingers and pulling gently on each toe,

---

* These games are courtesy of Chris Jackson. For a larger list of games, visit his subreddit "List of fun MDMA activities for romantic partners."

as well as bending toes back as far as they can go comfortably.

On the less kinky side, there is always the foot rub.

There are easy "69" variations for most of these activities, including toe sucking and foot rubs, so both partners can enjoy simultaneous pleasure. One fun game is "mirroring," with one partner taking the lead while the other mirrors their movements. Some users report feeling a kind of synesthesia while doing this, somehow mistaking their own actions as resulting in the pleasure they're feeling.

It goes without saying that cleanliness is crucial.

### Ice

Apply directly to skin in sensitive areas: Ice the nipples; add crushed ice to the mouth for a radically different oral sex experience; chew ice and make out; ice up hands before a hand job or fingering; ice the lips before kissing; let a small piece of ice melt in the belly button or the small of the back, or on the soles of the feet.

### Kissing Lessons

It can be great fun when one partner plays the role of "never been kissed" while the other gives their inexperienced "friend" a tutorial on how to make out. This is a great game for couples to learn each other's preferred kissing styles. Take it further by pretending to be strictly platonic friends who slowly discover their repressed feelings for each other during the tutorial.

### Massage

A must-try on Ecstasy. Key areas include the scalp, face, neck, shoulders, back, butt, hands, and feet. Avoid the belly, but everywhere else is great. You do not need to be a professional.

Simply being lovingly touched and rubbed is divine. A gently scented massage oil is a must.

*Note:* This is not a good time to try deep tissue or other types of massage that could lead to soreness and bruising. Avoid using your elbows or other aggressive techniques.

### Trading Air

Try "trading air"—one partner inhales while the other exhales—for an intimate and curious sensation. Do not do this more than a few times consecutively, and stop immediately if either of you feels lightheaded.

Surround yourselves with pillows in the unlikely event of someone passing out, and if they do, relax; they'll bounce back as soon as they're breathing normally.

### Oral Sex Coaching

Most of us enjoy receiving oral sex, but the empathogen qualities of Ecstasy or ketamine can be valuable teachers to help us please our partners.

This game begins with one partner performing oral sex on the other in the position chosen by the recipient. The giver performs the act while the recipient watches, gently and encouragingly providing instruction. The recipient directs the giver on what to do and how to do it, using simple commands like *faster*, *slower*, *harder*, *softer*, and possibly gently using their hands to manipulate the giver's head.

### Shower/Bath

The sheer popularity of this activity puts it in the top-ten Ecstasy experiences and comes highly recommended.

If you have a handheld, adjustable showerhead, experiment with different settings in different places. Women report good things with the massaging pulse setting and both sexes enjoy the gentle pulsing on their buttholes. Use your imagination.

Try soaping each other up and sensually washing each other's bodies, shampooing each other's hair, and soaking in a warm bath with bubbles.

Hot tubs and swimming pools can also be fun, but beware of hot temps and the potential for drowning. Stay safe.

### Slip and Slide

Coat your bodies with your favorite lubricant or coconut oil and slide all over each other. Be advised that these oils can ruin fabrics, so use a play sheet or put down some towels or blankets you don't care about.

### Slow Dancing

While upbeat club dancing is all the "rave" when it comes to Ecstasy, the romantic slow dance gets much less play. Put on a love song you both enjoy and just hold each other close. You don't have to know how to dance; simply embracing and swaying to the music is euphoric.

### Smell

MDMA enhances all your senses, including smell. Many partners enjoy their partner's natural scent. Key areas include underarms, genitals, and feet. Ecstasy is a full-body experience. No reason to exclude your nose.

### Softie

Many men can't get or maintain an erection on psychedelics, but this shouldn't rule out oral sex. Men report great satisfaction and unique experience from the "softie"—oral stimulation of a flaccid penis.

There are quite a few oral tricks that really aren't options on an erect penis. Kissing, licking, sucking, and rolling the penis around in the mouth with an active tongue can be tantalizing for both partners.

### Eye Gazing

Look directly into each other's eyes for as long as you can without saying anything. You might be surprised by how intense this can be or by the smile you can't suppress. Some couples report laughter and other surprises.

### Tongue Play

Tongue sucking is generally reported as being one of the top-ten best Ecstasy experiences, even if it's not something you usually do. One partner sticks their tongue out as far as they comfortably can while the other partner takes it into their mouth, providing suction, tongue-on-tongue stimulation, and even working the tongue in and out of their mouth similar to a blow job.

Try sensually licking your partner's exposed tongue, on top and underneath, noting the different textures and feels.

Ask your partner to push their tongue against the roof of their mouth toward their front teeth, exposing the lingual frenulum, the thin strip of tissue that runs vertically from the floor of the mouth to the undersurface of the tongue. Lick it. There's a good chance this will be a new sensation for both of you.

People with tongue piercings report some unique joys related entirely to their body jewelry. Do be careful, as there have been incidents of people chewing their metal tongue jewelry and doing some damage. If you have metal in your mouth, we highly recommend substituting with softer tongue jewelry such as "bioplast" for the duration of the roll.

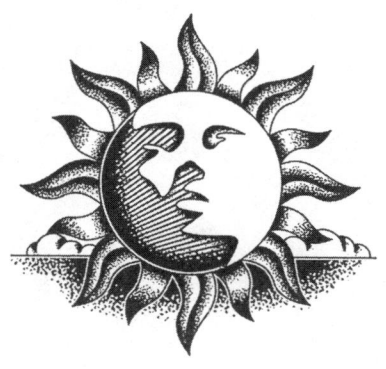

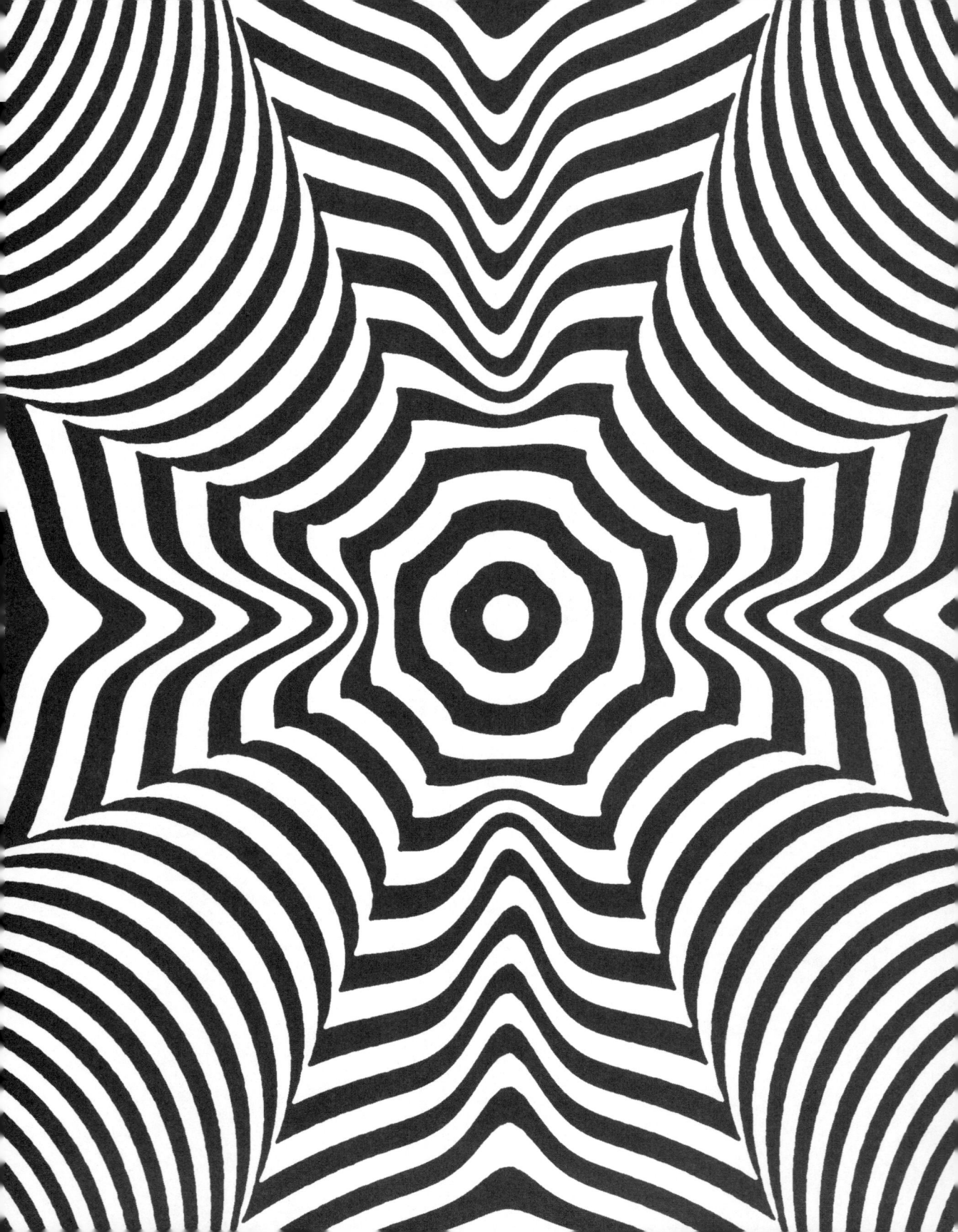

# CHAPTER 7

# HARM REDUCTION

## SPIRITUAL EMERGENCIES, PSYCHOLOGICAL EMERGENCIES, AND AVOIDING EMERGENCY ROOMS

H arm reduction is more than just a good thing to know about. It involves awareness of how to care for yourself and others, and how to avoid risks. The guiding principle is that it's better to arm people with information, including how to reduce risk, than to tell them not to engage in supposedly harmful behaviors. It gives people who use substances of any kind the tools and information to avoid psychological problems like isolation, confusion, or panic, and physical problems like infection or overdose, before they occur, and it helps them deal with problems if they do.

Harm reduction is centered on respect and compassion rather than coercion, scare tactics, or punishment. You don't need to be abstinent to practice harm reduction or receive services. It's not judgmental about drug use; nor is it substance-specific, which is why this chapter also includes information on non-psychedelic substances.

## Psychological Harm Reduction

By now you know that psychedelic experiences are not always positive, mystical, or spiritually illuminating. Even if you've followed best practices, journeys can leave you confused, shaken, and in some cases damaged in ways that are difficult to recover from. One of the many terrible side effects of prohibition is that it forces substances, research, and knowledge underground, and stifles the proliferation of that knowledge. This includes some of the lesser-known harms that are coming to light in these early days of the psychedelic renaissance. I'm raising these issues not to scare you, but to make you aware, so you don't feel isolated or panicked should a psychedelic/spiritual emergency occur.

A good number of these issues have been surfaced by Jules Evans, the founder of the *Ecstatic Integration* Substack series, which is devoted to highlighting underreported distress that sometimes accompanies psychedelic or spiritual journeys (including silent retreats and meditation).

Evans's first "spiritual emergency" occurred following an LSD trip he had at age eighteen, which left him destabilized and confused for years. A combination of psychiatric care, cognitive behavioral therapy, and Stoic philosophy helped him out of that hole.

When he was forty Evans returned to psychedelics, but rather than stepping in cautiously he dove in headfirst. He signed up for a ten-day, five-ceremony ayahuasca retreat in the Peruvian jungle. (Why he didn't start by attending just one local ceremony is a question that he is still asking himself.) His overall experience was satisfying, but in one ceremony he literally lost himself: He forgot his name and identity, and the fact that he was a human in a body. It terrified him, but he reconstituted.

Things spiraled downward once he left the retreat and found himself alone in the Galápagos Islands, where he went for his own self-styled form of integration. He had a powerful sense "that the reality I was in was not real." This state of dissociation is called derealization, and it occurs to more than a few people after psychedelics. Over the next weeks, Evans battled through an "ontological uncertainty" that left him cognitively disabled. He was unable to comprehend books (except, inexplicably and luckily, books by the Buddhist nun/writer Pema Chodron). Conversations confused him, which ratcheted up his social anxiety. He worried that his mind was going to be stuck in a permanent state of discombobulation, but none of these concerns came to bear. He had a soft landing.

Today, Evans is circumspect about his experiences. "I look at them as interesting. And maybe they were healing. A lot of people navigate these challenging experiences and eventually fold them into a better, more dimensional life."[1] He later learned that a family member was diagnosed with bipolar disorder, an unspoken family secret that might have changed his mind about returning to psychedelics had he known.

In conjunction with clinical psychologist Dr. Willoughby Britton and religious studies scholar Dr. Jared Lindahl, Evans has created a taxonomy of the holes people can fall into after journeys. They include:

- Anxiety and fear: Fear of going mad, fear of permanently damaging yourself, plus the social anxiety that may accompany such feelings.
- HPPD: Hallucinogen persisting perception disorder, a rare condition in which perceptual distortions continue for months or years after the trip. These were once known as flashbacks, and they occur more commonly in people who are red/green color-blind.
- Social disconnection from family, love, work, partner.
- Existential confusion: *What the hell was that? What did it mean? Who am I and where do I go from here?*
- Ego inflation: An ecstatic experience can create the illusion that you are a member of a spiritual elite, which can end up leaving you feeling alienated or isolated.
- Spiritual bypassing: This phrase was coined in 1980 by the psychotherapist and author John Welwood, who defined it as using "spiritual ideas and practices to sidestep personal, emotional 'unfinished business,' to shore up a shaky sense of self, or to ignore basic needs." In other words, avoidance, repression, or using your newfound spirituality to solidify the shaky ground beneath your feet.
- Spiritual euthanasia: Another common delusion in which you think that you and your fellow celebrants are holier than thou or more pure than the masses who aren't seeking spiritual elevation.
- Overfetishization of psychedelics: This can include escapist behaviors like

bouncing from festival to festival, retreat to retreat—always chasing the next peak experience. This form of escapism can also lead you to denigrate or undervalue everyday life.

- Loneliness: Any challenging psychedelic experience can leave you feeling isolated, especially if you don't have a community to hold you.
- And of course, heightened vulnerability can leave you prey to sketchy gurus, cults, and false messiahs, all of which are already showing up on the psychedelic landscape.

Many of the strategies to avoid boggling your own mind are covered in chapter 4: Engage a guide or sitter, factor in set and setting, plan ahead, integrate. Another crucial factor is dosing appropriately. For newbies, starting small can make all the difference—you can always take more, but you can't take less. Starting with a light dose is less likely to be overwhelming or challenging, and it can lay the foundation for stronger trips down the line. Navigating a reality-rattling experience and returning to earth in one piece will be easier if you work up to it gradually.

In many cases, going for the heroic dose may increase the psychological risks without necessarily adding benefit. Large quantities don't correlate with expanded insight, growth, or mystical/magical experience. Many users report having profound realizations, deepened connections with partners, and increased awe or wonder on low to moderate doses. Less can be more when mitigating psychological and physical risks. Using the lowest dose to achieve the desired effects is recommended, especially if you're new.

Should you find yourself struggling psychologically during or after a trip, there are a number of resources available. Support lines and therapist/counselor directories can be found at the end of this chapter.

## Physical Harm Reduction

You can't control your trip, but you can control what you put in your body. A shocking percentage of street drugs (12 to 15 percent of powdered stimulants[2] and up to 70 percent of counterfeit pills[3]) are now laced with fentanyl. Most psychedelics aren't usually a risk for fentanyl, but anything that comes as a pill or powder (notably MDMA) could be contaminated. Testing your drugs is the only way to ensure that they are free of fentanyl as well as xylazine or other substances that can harm or kill you.

Fentanyl may be the most severe risk, but it is by no means the only one. Pills, powders, liquids, and blotters can contain chemical

---

## WARNING: THE CHOCOLATE CHIP EFFECT

Once a pill is pressed, its components are locked in place. This is called the chocolate chip effect. Because fentanyl is rarely distributed evenly throughout the base powder, part of a pill might have no fentanyl, while another part has a lot. This is why testing just a portion of a pill will not assure you that the rest of the tablet is free of fentanyl. You must dissolve everything you plan to consume prior to testing.

---

adulterants in addition to the intended substance, or they can be a different drug altogether. This is most often true of MDMA sold in pill form, which commonly contains bulking agents, fillers, and/or other drugs such as caffeine, cocaine, amphetamine, DXM, and cathinones. Recent reports also indicate adulterants are showing up in over-the-counter magic mushroom chocolate bars and candies that are marketed as containing "proprietary mushroom nootropic blends."[4] Unknowingly consuming the wrong drugs can be unpleasant or disconcerting at best, and fatal at worst. Unintentionally taking multiple drugs at once can hugely increase risks and strain on the body.

## TESTING SUBSTANCES

An increasing number of chemicals are being sold as MDMA, LSD, and ketamine. The only way to know what you're about to ingest is to test. *Note:* BunkPolice.org recently released an app called Transparency Harm Reduction that provides excellent videos and instructions so you can learn to test your drugs, and, most importantly, read the results in the palm of your hand. See Resources for more information.

### Reagent Kits

Reasonably priced reagent testing kits are sold by DanceSafe, Bunk Police, and Grassroots Harm Reduction, among other such organizations.

### QTests

Reagent testing determines the presence of unwelcome drugs, but it does not determine purity or potency.

QTests, manufactured by the German company Miraculix, are sold by the US nonprofits Grassroots Harm Reduction and Bunk Police. These single-use tests are pricier at around $25.00 but they test for the concentration of active ingredients in your MDMA, LSD, psilocybin mushrooms, or cannabis flower.

*Note:* While the color tester is good, it's less accurate than a spectrometer. Make sure you read the sample against the whitest surface you can find (i.e., a white porcelain or ceramic plate).

### Test Strips

Over 150 people die every day from overdosing on fentanyl and synthetic opioids, according to the Centers for Disease Control. Even small doses of fentanyl can be deadly.

Fentanyl is impossible to see, taste, or smell and it is increasingly being found in cocaine and other street drugs.

Fentanyl test strips (FTS) have become useful tools to harm reduction. The most widely distributed FTS is the Rapid Response Test Strip manufactured by BTNX. These strips are designed to detect several common fentanyl analogs in urine but *they were not designed to test pills*, which makes them woefully inadequate for what's going on today.

DanceSafe, Bunk Police, and Grassroots Harm Reduction distribute fentanyl test strips that detect fentanyl in powders or pressed pills. They require the use of either a milligram scale or a 10 mg micro scoop.

Fentanyl test strips are also frequently available from community health centers, needle exchanges, and harm reduction booths.

*Important: Not all fentanyl test strips work the same.* DanceSafe, Bunk Police, and Grassroots Harm Reduction fentanyl test strips have been laboratory-assessed to work for harm reduction purposes, as opposed to just urine testing.

These new strips use a superior antibody that is more sensitive to fentanyl and its analogs. This means that unlike the Rapid Response strips, they won't produce false positives with MDMA, cocaine, or methadone, when used according to the instructions.

## CHOOSING A PSYCHEDELIC RETREAT: BUYER BEWARE

While there are beautiful and well-administered retreat centers in eye-poppingly beautiful places around the world, in this boom market there are also amateur operations run by self-styled gurus offering shoddy or little aftercare. Before you plonk down thousands of dollars for that dream ayahuasca retreat in the Peruvian jungle three hundred miles away from a paved road, or in a remote village where few people speak your language, there are some basic boxes that need to be ticked.

- Don't base any decisions on pretty pictures from websites or Instagram photos of happy beautiful people in ceremony.
- Don't go on any retreat without speaking to the organizers in person to ask questions.
- Have the organizers asked you to fill out a detailed medical history that includes current and past medications along with your history of mental illness and that of your family? If they haven't, beware.

  If they have, be sure to answer the questions truthfully. Some centers will work with you, but they likely won't accept liability for injury. Being clear about your condition helps to ensure your well-being, the longevity of the center, and the longevity of the

psychedelic movement in general.
- If something goes wrong—and lots can go wrong, even in paradise (see the box below)—is there a doctor on call? Where is the nearest hospital? Is reliable transportation always available?

## SEXUAL AND MENTAL ABUSE AND TRANSGRESSIONS

Psychedelic therapy, whether with MDMA or ayahuasca, can lead people into sketchy ethical territory. There is a huge imbalance of power between therapist/guide and client during sessions; some people may already have existing mental health issues, which, coupled with high doses of a psychedelic, can lead unethical practitioners to exploit their vulnerabilities.

Ever since psychedelic therapy began in the 1970s, there have been reports of sexual abuse between professionals and clients; the most infamous and disturbing recent example occurred in the highly controlled 2015 MAPS Phase III trial of MDMA for PTSD.[5] Since then, MAPS has publicly issued a code of ethical conduct for guides and therapists.

Nonconsensual sex is a no-go. It's difficult to determine just how widespread it is in the psychedelic community. Be sure to have the consent conversation before signing up for any psychedelic experience.

- Who are the leaders? What are their credentials or experience? ("I've taken four hundred ayahuasca journeys" is not enough, sorry.)
- Do they provide a full itinerary of what to expect?
- How many celebrants does the retreat host at one time? Some retreats serve sixty people, which sounds to me like an assembly-line operation. If it sounds the same to you, keep searching.
- Aftercare: Is there any? What is it and for how long? Some retreats end the day of the last ceremony. After all the hugs goodbye, you could find yourself dropped off at some airport feeling hyper-receptive, a bit lost, and ill-equipped to return to modern life. It's always wise to plan some aftercare following your retreat.
- And no, it's not cool for the retreat operators to ask for your bank card and PIN so they can run to the ATM "just in case you need something during the ceremony." Trust me, it has happened!

I know, that sounds like a lot, but there are a growing number of reports from people who have had identity-shattering experiences on retreats. If you have any doubts, don't go. A week on a beach may be the better option.

---

## DON'T GO OFF YOUR PSYCHIATRIC MEDS TO ATTEND A RETREAT

*Warning:* Tapering off any antidepressant or psychiatric medication should be done only under medical supervision, and it can take months. Many "experts" suggest quitting meds eight weeks before a journey. Nonsense! Each body is different, the length of time you've been on the meds affects the taper, and quitting them too quickly can leave you seriously destabilized.

*Warning:* People with certain heart conditions should not sit in ceremony with any substance, in particular ibogaine. A frank talk with your trusted medical providers is in order.

# EVEN IN FIRST CLASS, THINGS CAN GO WRONG!

I attended a high-end weeklong psilocybin retreat in Jamaica in exchange for a portion of my consulting fee with a psychedelic company based in New York City. I know the leaders personally, and they take their work as hosts and facilitators very seriously. Before being accepted, I went through in-depth medical screening. Three preparatory meetings were arranged before leaving New York to set individual intentions for the journey, and every detail, from transportation to and from the Montego Bay airport to each person's dietary needs, was accounted for. Upon arriving in our rooms, each of the celebrants was presented with their own journal accompanied by a personal note written by the organizer based on those intention-setting explorations. We knew we were in exquisite care.

The food was delicious and the accommodations sumptuous; the music was sung and played live. Massages were on offer. Each of the three guides had been practicing for years. On the last of three psilocybin journeys, I confidently swallowed a heroic dose. Takeoff was easy, but at some point—midway through the trip?—I sat up and the world lurched out of balance. It was as if I was flying in an airplane that suddenly dropped a thousand feet in the air. Dizzy and spinning, I felt as if the core of my being had been hollowed out. I laid my head down to wait it out, *except it didn't end.*

Once the ceremony concluded, everyone in the group of ten ambled upstairs to view the luminous night sky, but I was unable to raise my body off my mat without spinning. John, the primary space holder, kept me company, playing great tracks and maintaining a watchful eye. Eventually he helped me to my feet, but I was wobbly and unable to maintain balance. John escorted me to my room and into my bed, which unfortunately began to whirl when I opened my eyes. He wanted to summon the doctor. I declined, preferring instead to sleep it off.

In the morning, the sunlight was blinding. The room was gyrating such that I had to crawl to the bathroom. I was unable to stand to pee and I wobbled on the toilet seat. In my fuzzy cognition I wondered if I was the first man in history to have scrambled his brain with psilocybin. *Was I going to be permanently off-balance?*

That afternoon, my partner, who is a physical therapist, called and surmised that I had vertigo. Somehow, be it through flying or swimming (or taking psilocybin, I feared), the calcium crystals in my inner ear that maintain equilibrium got thrown out of whack. He sent me a YouTube video on the Epley maneuver, which I shared with one of the guides. Luckily for me she also happened to be a nurse practitioner and was soon manipulating my head to jostle my inner ear crystals back into place. Without my

*CONTINUED*

asking, the retreat leaders kindly arranged for me to stay in my room an extra night after the other guests departed, and then accompanied me to the airport the following day just in case. That was a great comfort and far beyond the call of duty.

Vertigo turned out to be a short-lived problem with no further consequences, but let me assure you that those first few hours of confusion and fear with no end in sight served as a stark reminder that even in first class, things can go wrong!

### IF YOU'RE HAVING A BAD TRIP AND NEED TO TALK . . .

Staffed by trained volunteers who understand what you're going through, the Fireside Project is open every day from 11 AM to 11 PM PST. They also maintain an active presence at many festivals including Burning Man, Outside Lands, and Mycologia.

If you're tripping or need to process a past trip, or if you're a tripsitter who needs a hand, Fireside Project volunteers are trained to get you through any tough time by offering "real time support for those times when time just doesn't seem real."

Keep their number in your phone: 62-Fireside, or download their free app.

*Note:* This emotional support service is strictly nonclinical/nonmedical. Callers should use 911 or 988 in the event of an emergency. Firesideproject.org

## Harm Reduction and Education Resources

### DanceSafe

If you've been to a well-organized rave, festival, or big music event in the last thirty years, you've probably come across DanceSafe's booths—those places where you'll find helpful non-judgy volunteers to help you test your pills and powders. (This is an essential healthcare service that IMHO the government should be providing.) On their website you can also buy test strips that allow you to home test your drugs for the presence of nasty adulterants like fentanyl or Xylazine. Bonus: Their easy-to-read instructions come in English and Spanish. DanceSafe also sells reagent kits (more complicated to use) that tell you if the contents of your drugs are not what you think they are. Their Instagram is full of bitesize drug info that we should all know (but frequently forget). DanceSafe.org

### The Bunk Police

The Bunk Police is another excellent resource center that sells all manner of drug testing supplies. The group has recently released a free and super-useful AI-powered app called Transparency Harm Reduction that shows users how to use testing kits for most substances all in one place on your phone. Bonus: The app has over a thousand lab-verified spot kit videos that show you exactly what your drug reaction should look like. BunkPolice.com

### Grassroots Harm Reduction

In 2024, Emanuel Sferios, the founder of DanceSafe, had philosophical disagreements

# ESSENTIAL HARM REDUCTION TOOL KIT

Don't trip without these essential items.

## Digital Scale
Milligram scales are essential for accurately measuring the doses of your drugs.

## Micro Scoop
If you don't have a milligram scale, a micro scoop is a convenient tool that measures 10 mg of any crushed powder.

## Earplugs
Harm reduction includes keeping your body safe. Loud music for extended periods of time can cause hearing damage, so it's never a bad idea to use earplugs. DanceSafe-branded earplugs are engineered to allow in all frequencies at just the right level. They fit comfortably and deliver clear sound. Bonus: They come with a spare third earplug if one gets lost. (One *always* does.)

## Pill Cutter
With certain drugs, "less is more" can make a huge difference. Pill cutters help you lower your dose by easily cutting pressed tablets in half with minimal breakage.

## Sniffer
If you choose to snort, always use your own device! Why? When snorted substances come into contact with the lining of the nasal cavity, blood vessels in your nose can dilate and break. This can allow microscopic amounts of blood to leak onto the snorting device. If this blood is infected with hepatitis C or other diseases, there is a risk of transmission. Cut your own straws or splurge on DanceSafe's aluminum straws that come in different disco colors.

## Hydration Pack
Dehydration is one of the main causes of medical tent visits during festivals, so drink water! If you're one who doesn't want to carry a bottle, DanceSafe offers a "WeLoveConsent"-branded 1.5-liter pack that keeps you hydrated while spreading the message of consent within the music and nightlife communities.

## Roll Kit
Bunk Police offers a handy pack of vitamins and minerals for MDMA recovery that includes Vitamin C, Green Tea Extract, ALA, CoEnzyme Q10 and other supplements. There's no guarantee that they help recovery, but they won't hurt.

with the future direction of the nonprofit he launched in 1998, so he peeled away to launch a new organization that operates on a less centralized, more localized model. GRHR's online shop sells fentanyl strips and reagents; it is also the main US supplier of QTests that measure the potency of mushrooms, LSD, MDMA, and cannabis. GRHR offers guidance, training, and educational materials to local groups that are dedicated to doing peer-to-peer harm reduction in their communities. All profits are turned into microgrants to member organizations. GrassRootsHarmReduction.org

### Drugs and Me

Upon first glance, I thought this was just a blog, but this organization offers accurate information on a wide scope of drugs including psychedelics. They combine anecdotal experience with scientific research and present it in a user-friendly format. This is a good resource for easy-to-digest facts about drugs as well as more specific and personal accounts of other people's experiences. Drugs and Me is London based but operates internationally. Drugsand.me

### Zendo Project
### *Psychedelic Harm Redux Manual*

The Zendo Project *Psychedelic Harm Reduction Manual* was created by Burning Man participants who volunteer to support people undergoing difficult psychedelic experiences. The Zendo Project seeks to turn those experiences into opportunities for learning and personal growth, and to reduce the number of drug-related hospitalizations. The manual was written in 2013 for guests at Burning Man, so the logistical information can be ignored. But it remains a thorough, useful—and free—guide to harm reduction best practices.

https://zendoproject.org/manuals/manual-of-psychedelic-support/

### Erowid

Erowid is one of the oldest and most comprehensive online resources for information on psychoactive substances. Started by the couple Earth and Fire Erowid, this site hosts a massive and at first glance unwieldy database of user experience reports, as well as information on legality, culture, spirituality, and science. Erowid.org

### DrugsData

DrugsData (formerly EcstasyData) is the independent drug-checking program of the Erowid Center. Its purpose is to collect, review, manage, and publish testing results from their lab and other analysis projects worldwide. DrugsData offers paid, anonymous, nonquantitative testing of all psychoactive drugs through their DEA-licensed laboratory. Find their price list as well as instructions on how to send them a sample for testing on their website. Results are posted confidentially fourteen to twenty-one days after the lab receives the sample. Drugsdata.org

### Psychedelic Support

Psychedelic Support offers education and support around psychedelics. In addition to courses and trainings on psychedelics, harm reduction, and best practices, they curate a MAPS-approved directory of licensed mental health providers trained in psychedelic therapy. While providers cannot offer psychedelic therapy outside of clinical trials, this is a great resource for preparation, integration, or coping with difficult experiences. Psychedelic.support

### TripSit

TripSit is a harm reduction and education site, promoting "discourse from scientific, medical, and philosophical angles." They offer guides on harm reduction, tripsitting, recovery, dosing, as well as their own wiki with info pages for many different substances. TripSit.me

### Bluelight

Bluelight is primarily an online forum with nearly a half million members and around four hundred thousand threads on trip reports, drug culture, art, education, harm reduction, and many other related topics. Bluelight partners with researchers around the world, providing content for studies and helping to design and spread surveys through their network. Bluelight.org

### MAPS

The Multidisciplinary Association for Psychedelic Studies (MAPS) is the most important organization on the front lines of psychedelic research and legalization. Started in 1986, this nonprofit has raised over $140 million for research and education. Look here for information about ongoing clinical trials on marijuana, MDMA, LSD, ibogaine, and ayahuasca. MAPS.org

### PsychonautWiki

This Wikipedia-style resource offers wiki pages on pretty much any psychedelic drug you can think of, as well as information on meditation, lucid dreaming, sensory deprivation, and extraction tutorials. This is a comprehensive resource for dosing and safety information and it includes thorough lists of all possible subjective effects for each substance. Psychonautwiki.org

### Energy Control

Energy Control is a confidential drug testing service based in Barcelona and other locations throughout Spain. To have your drugs tested, you must first fill out a form; once approved, they will send you further instructions on how to complete payment and ship your sample for testing. Price varies based on the substance being tested and results can take seven to twenty-one business days. There is currently no US branch, but the drug testing service is open to all international customers. EnergyControl-International.org

### ICEERS Support Center

For those going through difficult processes with psychoactive plants, ICEERS support sessions are free of charge and are conducted by trained professionals with expertise in psychedelic assistance. The service is a complement to—but not a replacement for—medical, psychological, or psychiatric attention; it is best used for post-trip integration. The only way to reach them is via a request form on their website. They attend to inquiries according to availability, giving priority to the gravest cases. Sessions are in English or Spanish and last forty-five to sixty minutes. Staffing is limited, and typical response time is one or two days. ICEERS is based in Barcelona. Iceers.org/support-center-2

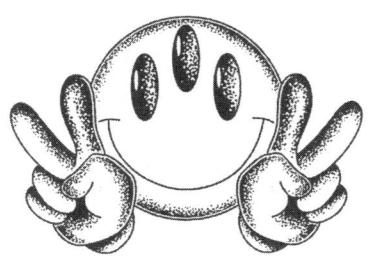

# Afterword

--------------------------------

## THE FOOTHILLS OF DISCOVERY:
## YOUR ROLE IN THE PSYCHEDELIC RESURGENCE

*We are at a historic moment. Old social orders are rapidly changing.*
*Economic powers are restructuring for the future. There is widespread*
*popular interest in the brain and the mind as never before.*
*Interest in research with psychedelics seems to be growing....*

You might think that the statement above was written today but it was, lamentably, written over thirty years ago in 1993 by David Nichols as he was launching the Heffter Research Institute. While I hope to end this book on an optimistic note, I can't do so without reminding you, dear readers, that we've been here before, several times in fact. Today's psychedelic boom is also an echo of the past. While the leaders in the psychedelic movement agree among themselves that the world is finally on the path to recognizing the benefits of these substances, there's no guarantee that it won't go off the rails. So let's get it right this time. Everyone has a role to play. Here are ten ways you can pitch in.

1.  Tell your story.

    When a bill for legalizing medical marijuana was on the ballot in California in 1995, organizers learned that the best way to change minds wasn't through advertising or arguing. It was through sharing personal stories. Even hardened opponents of cannabis legalization were more likely to be swayed when someone they knew told them how using the plant alleviated their suffering. Polling today says the same is true with psychedelics. So come out! Summon your courage and tell your story, especially to people who may not want to hear it.

2.  Don't preach.

    Breathless, frothing headlines accompany every boom. It happened with the advent of the internet, it's happening with AI, and it's happening with psychedelics. So when you do tell your story, tell the full story. Bad things can happen. There are real risks. Not everyone should use psychedelics. Keep it real. Stay humble. Psychedelics are not a religion, so don't preach.

3.  Arm yourself with facts.

    Ayahuasca won't save your life (but it may provide insight on what you can do to change your life).

    Tripping on MDMA at a rave won't end your PTSD (but clinical studies show that

MDMA-assisted therapy reverses PTSD for 70 percent of subjects).

Mushrooms won't heal your depression (but the FDA is fast-tracking psilocybin-assisted therapy for treatment-resistant depression).

There is a real power to under-promising and over-delivering. The less you promise and the more facts you offer, the more persuasive you and your story will be.

4.  Be ready to contend with (and integrate) opposition.

Listen, and try not to argue with people who don't agree with you. Everyone responds better when they feel heard. By the way, opposition creates an opportunity to discuss what the future could look like. Legalization efforts will have a better chance to succeed if they include support programs for people who have bad experiences while tripping, programs for integration or peer group counseling, help lines, and research into what works best to help folks through tough experiences. Oregon legalized all drug use without having support in place, and state officials were surprised when overdoses shot up. Let's not repeat that.

5.  Think beyond medicine.

At the moment, the psychedelic conversation is focused on treating medical conditions. Alleviating suffering is essential, but along with that we need conversations about how to manage production and distribution for recreational users. The days of buying a bag of mysterious white powder with no quality control should end, and not a minute too soon.

Governments and regulatory bodies need smart policies for smart and safer use. At the same time, we need more discussions and clarity on how psychedelics can be used for human flourishing.

6.  Volunteer or build a career.

If and when federal legalization moves forward, the need for experts in policy, counseling, technology, and palliative care will skyrocket. Even now, as more states and municipalities legalize psychedelic-assisted therapy, the demand for therapists far exceeds supply. If the idea of becoming a psychedelic-assisted therapist piques your interest, get trained now.

7.  Get credentialed.

If you are in school, get your degree. You'll have more credibility if you can demonstrate that you have the discipline and stamina to get an advanced degree and contend with the inevitable bureaucracy endemic to both the academic and scientific establishments.

8.  Register to vote.

Even if you're disaffected by politics, don't dismiss the power of your vote. Voters moved the needle on ballot issues in Oregon and Colorado. More statewide ballot initiatives are coming. You can also talk to your own town's police and legislators about making psychedelic possession the lowest enforcement priority.

9.  Support organizations that support the whole human.

If you're thinking of trying ketamine treatment, choose clinics that offer therapy rather than ones that do just an IV drip. It's better for you and better for therapists who will share some of the proceeds. Johnson & Johnson makes more money when you use esketamine without engaging therapeutic support because you'll buy more of their product.

10. Fund the future, if you can.

If you have some money, consider supporting nonprofit psychedelic research organizations such as the Usona Institute, the Beckley Foundation, Breaking Convention, The Chacruna Institute, VETS, or MAPS—organizations that benefit the many, not just the few.

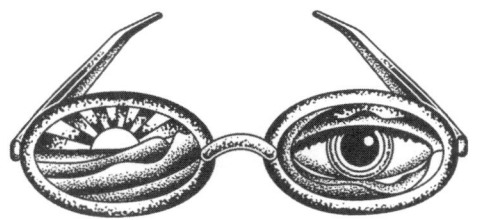

# Acknowledgments

Deep thanks and gratitude to all the brilliant, brave, and beautiful people who took time to share their expertise, wisdom, experiences, and thoughts with me:

Julie Holland, Gül Dölen, James Fadiman, Jeffrey Guss, Rick Doblin and the staff at MAPS, Erica Zelfand, Ben Sessa, Hamilton Morris, Paul Stamets, Leonard Pickard, Rick Strassman, Jonathan Dickinson, Emanuel Sferios, Julia Christina Reibelt, Ido Cohen, Juan, Allison Wells, Leonardo Vando, Rachel Harris, Matthew Johnson, Zach Walsh, Manesh Girn, Robert Bray, Erik Davis, Tom Kingsley Brown, Vincente Alonso, Kristie Jacobsen, Amanda Elo'Esh, Elyse Raupp-Gardner, Norman Ohler, Chris Jackson, Marcus and Amber Capone, Mario Garnier, Reilly Capps, Dylan Beynon, Jules Evans, Jason Silva, Jamie Wheal, the fine folks at Qualia Research Initiative, Madison Margolin and Shelby Hartman, publishers of *DoubleBlind* magazine, Fire and Ice Erowid, the brains behind ICEERS, and to Tim Ferriss, Andrew Huberman, and Third Wave podcasts, all of whom have shone the light on the science and history of psychedelics.

Special thanks to Dante Ascarrunz for his smarts and his stamina in helping me to research and refine this book, to Cody Gibbons, chemistry wizard, to Adriana Kertzer for her legal advice and overall enthusiasm, and to Kat Lakey and the Psychedelic Assembly in New York City for providing shelter, coffee, and a pleasant place to work.

The fine humans at Black Dog & Leventhal: Becky Koh, Katie Benezra, Melanie Gold, Kate Karol, Brenna Franzitta, and Joe Davidson all helped turn 90,000 words into a lovely printed object, and Mark Gottlieb made the deal happen.

To my friends who provided steadfast emotional consultation and consolation: Karen Rinaldi, Nick Hyman, the Cardea Clan—Ross Ellenhorn, Dimitri Murgianis, Zach Reick, Jill Reick, Aisha Delfaus, Paige Rothaus, John Maclean/The Juan Maclean—Sarah Siskind, and Nick Gillespie.

And to Kevin Lindsay, the rock in my life, who keeps me tethered, warmly embraced, and feeling younger each day.

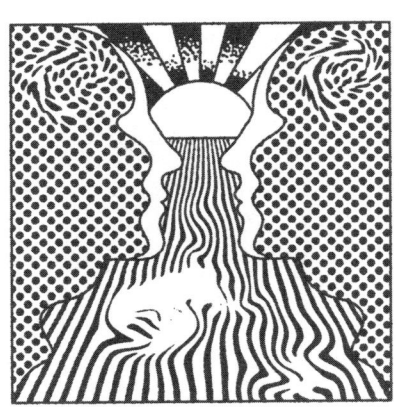

# Notes

----------------

**Author's Note**

1. Bienemann, Stomato Ruschel, Campos, et al., 2020.
2. Fadiman, 2011, p. 62.

**1. Welcome to the Psychedelic Resurgence**

1. Krebs and Johansen, 2013.ron
2. Hofmann, 1976.

**2. Birth, Ban, Boom!**

1. ICEERS, "San Pedro: Basic Info," https://www.iceers.org/san-pedro-basic-info/.
2. Shroder, 2014.
3. Hofmann, 1976.
4. Hofmann, 1979, p. 21.
5. Ohler, 2024, p. 35.
6. Hofmann, 1979, p. 22.
7. Ohler, 2024, p. 69.
8. Pellerin, 1998, p. 46.
9. Lattin, 2012.
10. Doblin, 1991.
11. Doblin, 2021.
12. Langlitz, 2012, p. 32.
13. Weil, 2019.
14. Johnson, n.d.
15. *LSD in the United States*, 1995, p. 8; Morris, 2010.
16. Morris and Ash, 2010.
17. Morris, 2010.
18. Nichols, 2018.
19. Griffiths, Richards, McCann, et al., 2006.
20. NAMI, "Mental Health by the Numbers," n.d.
21. Edakubo and Fushimi, 2020.
22. Johnson, n.d.
23. Canadian Institutes of Health Research, 2023.
24. Virdi, 2020; UNC School of Medicine, 2020.
25. Grand View Research, Mushroom Market Analysis Report and Forecasts for 2022–2030. https://www.grandviewresearch.com/industry-analysis/mushroom-market/.
26. Browne, 2023.
27. Sessa, 2016.
28. Sala, 2016.

**3. Under the Hood**

1. Waldman, 2017, p. 41.
2. Preller, Razi, Zeidman, et al., 2019.
3. Edsinger and Dölen, 2018.
4. Nardou, Sawyer, Song, et al., 2023.
5. Nardou, Sawyer, Song, et al., 2023.
6. Merabet, Maguire, Warde, et al., 2004.
7. Olson, 2023.
8. Sewell, Halpern, and Pope, 2006; Karst, Halpern, Bernateck, et al., 2010.

## 4. Have a Great Trip

1. Hartogsohn, 2020.
2. Barrett, 2020.
3. Lett, 2024.
4. Fadiman, 2011, p. 34.
5. Synthesis Institute, 2021.
6. Muraresku, 2021.
7. Fadiman, 2011, p. 37.

## The Substances: MDMA

1. Shulgin and Shulgin, 1991, p. 737.
2. Grinspoon and Doblin, 2001.
3. Eisner, 1989, p. 70.
4. Boyle and Connor, 2010.
5. Zelfand, 2024.
6. Reneman, Lavalaye, Schmand, et al., 2001.
7. "Dose-Effects Relationship for MDMA from Analyzed Samples," EROWID, 2011, https://erowid.org/chemicals/show_image.php?i=mdma/mdma_effects_curve_dims__i2016e0054_disp.jpg.
8. Zemishlany, Aizenberg, and Weizman, 2001.
9. Huberman, 2023.
10. Passie, 2018.
11. Passie, 2018.
12. Nuwer, "How MDMA Became the Club Drug of the Century," 2023.
13. Business Research Insights, EDM Industry Analysis Report and Forecasts for 2020–2032, 2024. https://www.businessresearchinsights.com/market-reports/edm-market-117946.
14. Passie, 2018.
15. Nuwer, "Understanding MDMA," 2023.
16. "Pure Ecstasy," 2015.
17. Mithoefer, Wagner, Mithoefer, et al., 2011.
18. MAPS, 2017.
19. Dumont, Sweep, van der Steen, et al., 2009.
20. Huberman, 2023.
21. Bedi, Phan, Angstadt, et al., 2009.
22. Singleton, Wang, Mithoefer, et al., 2023.
23. Nicholas, Wang, Coker, et al., 2022.
24. Sessa, Sakal, O'Brien, et al., 2019.
25. Danforth, Grob, Struble, et al., 2018.
26. Holland, 2001, p. 288.
27. Christie, Yazar-Klosinski, Nosova, et al., 2022.
28. Adamson, Metzner, and Catell, 2013, p. 187.
29. McNeil Jr., 2003.
30. Halpern, Sherwood, Hudson, et al., 2011.

## The Substances: Magic Mushrooms (Psilocybin /Psilocin)

1. Winkelman, 2019.
2. Fadiman, 2021.
3. Winkelman, 2019.
4. Griffiths, Richards, McCann, et al., 2006.
5. Gerber, García Flores, Ruiz, et al., 2021.
6. Gukasyan, Davis, Barrett, et al., 2022.
7. Gukasyan, Davis, Barrett, et al., 2022.
8. Ross, Bossis, Guss, et al., 2016.
9. Griffiths, Johnson, Carducci, et al., 2016.
10. Bogenschutz, Ross, Bhatt, et al., 2022.
11. Johnson, Garcia-Romeu, Cosimano, et al., 2014.
12. Johnson, Garcia-Romeu, and Griffiths, 2016.
13. Griffiths, Hurwitz, Davis, et al., 2019.
14. Brasher, 2022.

## The Substances: Ketamine

1. Rosenbaum, Gupta, Patel, et al., 2024; PsychonautWiki, "Ketamine," https://psychonautwiki.org/wiki/Ketamine; Drugs and Me, "Ketamine," https://www.drugsand.me/drugs/ketamine/.
2. Orhurhu, Vashisht, Claus, et al., 2024.
3. Reddit, "Ketamine Addiction," https://www.reddit.com/r/Ketamineaddiction/.
4. Silman, 2019.
5. Silman, 2019.
6. Silman, 2019.

7. https://www.reddit.com/r/ketamine/comments/wtc9qo/how_long_does_a_k_hole_last/.

8. Silman, 2019.

9. Ketamine for Mental Health, "Orientation Guide," https://ketamine therapyformental health.com/orientation_guide/.

10. Price, 2022; Price, Spotts, Panny, et al., 2022.

11. Hull, Malgaroli, Gazzaley, et al., 2022.

12. Institute for Quality and Efficiency in Health Care (IQWig), 2024.

13. Alemi, Min, Yousefi, et al., 2021.

14. Silman, 2019.

15. Ezquerra-Romano, Lawn, Krupitsky, et al., 2018.

16. Hu, 2024.

## The Substances: DMT/5-MeO-DMT

1. Barker, 2022.

2. Small Pharma Ltd., 2024.

3. Drugs and Me, "DMT," https://www.drugsand.me/drugs/dmt/; https://psychonautwiki.org/wiki/DMT; https://dancesafe.org/dmt/.

4. Strassman, 2012, p. 17.

5. Reddit, "DMT: My First Trip" (comments), https://www.reddit.com/r/DMT/comments/17x7xo1/my_first_trip/.

6. Strassman, 2022, p. 109.

7. Sklerov, Levine, Moore, et al., 2005.

8. Strassman, 2012, pp. 52–53.

9. Sample, 2023.

10. PsychonautWiki, "Changa," https://psychonautwiki.org/wiki/Changa.

11. Ortiz Bernal, Raison, Lancelotta, et al., 2022.

12. Five, "5-MeO-DMT Information," https://five-meo.education/basic-information/.

13. Uthaug, Lancelotta, Van Oorsouw, et al., 2019.

14. Davis, So, Lancelotta, et al., 2019.

15. Davis, Averill, Sepeda, et al., 2020.

16. Reckweg, van Leeuwen, Henquet, et al., 2023.

17. Sherwood, Claveau, and Lancelotta, 2020.

18. Pollan, 2018, p. 278.

19. Uthaug, Lancelotta, Van Oorsouw, et al., 2019.

20. Davis and Weil, 1992.

## The Substances: Ayahuasca

1. Schultes, Evans, Hofmann, et al., 1998, p. 124.

2. McKenna, 2007, pp. 21–44.

3. Grob, McKenna, Callaway, et al., 1996.

4. Bouso, González, Fondevila, et al., 2012.

5. Ruffell, Crosland-Wood, Palmer, et al., 2023.

6. Callaway, 1998, pp. 367–9.

7. Morales-García, de la Fuente Revenga, Alonso-Gil, et al., 2017.

8. Katchborian-Neto, Santos, Vilas-Boas, et al., 2022.

9. Plotkin, 2024.

## The Substances: LSD

1. Sala, 2016.

2. Johnson, Richards, and Griffiths, 2008.

3. Ohler, 2024, p. 102.

4. Kinzer, 2019.

5. Zeifman, Singhal, Breslow, et al., 2021.

6. "MindMed Receives FDA Breakthrough Therapy Designation," 2024.

7. Sewell, Halpern, and Pope Jr., 2006.

8. Karst, Halpern, Bernateck, et al., 2010.

9. "Weil says LSD cured his allergy," 2001.

10. Molla, Lee, Tare, et al., 2024.

11. Whitaker-Azmitia, 1999.

12. Markoff, 2006, p. xix.

13. Gandy, Bonelle, Jacobs, et al., 2002.

14. Rees, 2004.

15. Park, 2019.

16. Davis, 2024, p. 39.

17. Cohen, 2017.

**The Substances: Peyote/Mescaline/Huachuma**

1. Amazon Conservation Team, 2018.
2. Halpern, Sherwood, Hudson, et al., 2005.
3. Bergman, 1971.
4. Wallace, 1959.
5. ScienceDirect, "Neuroscience: Mescaline," https://www.sciencedirect.com/topics/neuroscience/mescaline.
6. Jay, "What Happened to Mescaline?", 2019; Huxley, 1954, p. 28.
7. ICEERS, "Peyote: Basic Info," https://www.iceers.org/peyote-basic-info/.
8. Dasgupta, 2019.
9. Winstock, Barratt, Ferris, et al., n.d.
10. Breen, 2024.
11. Golden, 2022.
12. Agin-Liebes, Haas, Lancelotta, et al., 2021.
13. ICEERS, "Peyote: Basic Info," https://www.iceers.org/peyote-basic-info/; PsychonautWiki, "Mescaline," https://psychonautwiki.org/wiki/Mescaline.
14. Huxley, 1954, p. 5.
15. Jay, "What Happened to Mescaline?", 2019.
16. Jay, "What Happened to Mescaline?", 2019.
17. Ogunbodede, McCombs, Trout, et al., 2010.
18. Hofmann and Schultes, 1979, p. 159.
19. Heaven, 2013, p. 5.
20. Jay, "What Happened to Mescaline?", 2019.
21. McConnell, 2024.

**The Substances: Ibogaine/Iboga**

1. Kentucky Attorney General, 2023.
2. Brown and Alper, 2018.
3. Mash, 2022.
4. Noller, Frampton, and Yazar-Klosinski, 2018.
5. Cherian, Keynan, Anker, et al., 2024.
6. Cable, 2024.
7. Dickinson, 2022.
8. Mash, 2022.

9. Kentucky Attorney General, 2023.
10. Mash, 2023.
11. Alper, Stajić, and Gill, 2012.
12. Rich, 2021.
13. Pinchbeck, 2003.
14. DeRienzo, 2005.
15. De Loenen, 2004.

**The Substances: Psychedelic Supplements**

1. Kilham, 2006.
2. Kilham, 2006.
3. Smorin, 2021.
4. "Kratom," 2022.
5. Holler, Vorce, McDonough-Bender, et al., 2011; TripSit Factsheet: "Kratom," tripsit.me/factsheets/Kratom.
6. Dubley, n.d.
7. Weiss, "This legal supplement," 2020.
8. Manganyi, Bezuidenhout, Regnier, et al., 2021.
9. Manganyi, Bezuidenhout, Regnier, et al., 2021.
10. Weiss, "Is cacao a psychoactive substance?", 2020.

**5. Microdosing**

1. Waldman, 2017, p. 49.
2. Waldman, 2017, p. 42.
3. Cavanna, Muller, de la Fuente, et al., 2022.
4. Rootman, Kiraga, Kryskow, et al., 2022.
5. Ramaekers, Hutten, Mason, et al., 2021.
6. Haijen, Hurks, and Kuypers, 2024.
7. Fadiman, 2019.
8. Calder and Hasler, 2023.
9. Lai, Naidu, Sabaratnam, et al., 2013.
10. Gasperi, Sibilano, Savini, et al., 2019.
11. Ma, Shen, Yu, et al., 2010.
12. Zhang, An, Hu, et al., 2016.

## 6. Couples and Psychedelics

1. Passie, 2018.
2. Ferriss, 2019.
3. van der Kolk, 2021.
4. Joshi, 2022.
5. Hanna and Thyssen, 2002.
6. Zemishlany, Aizenberg, and Weizman, 2001.
7. Peugh and Belenko, 2001.
8. Tiefer, 2006.

## 7. Harm Reduction

1. Evans, 2024.
2. Wagner, Fiuty, Page, et al., 2023.
3. "One Pill Can Kill," n.d.
4. Wright, 2024.
5. Rosin, 2022.

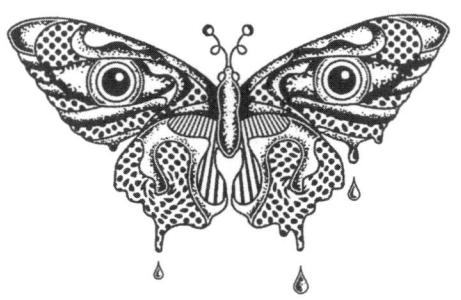

# Bibliography

Adamson, Sophia, Ralph Metzner, and Padma Catell. *Through the Gateway of the Heart.* Solarium Press, 2013.

Agin-Liebes G, Haas TF, Lancelotta R, et al. "Naturalistic Use of Mescaline Is Associated with Self-Reported Psychiatric Improvements and Enduring Positive Life Changes." *ACS Pharmacology & Translational Science* 4, no. 2 (March 2021): 543–52. https://doi.org/10.1021/acsptsci.1c00018.

Aixala, Marc. *Psychedelic Integration: Psychotherapy for Non-Ordinary States of Consciousness.* Synergetic Press, 2022.

Alemi F, Min H, Yousefi M, et al. "Effectiveness of common antidepressants: a post market release study." *EClinicalMedicine* 41, no. 101171 (October 25, 2021). https://doi.org/10.1016/j.eclinm.2021.101171.

Alper KR, Stajić M, Gill JR. "Fatalities temporally associated with the ingestion of ibogaine." *Journal of Forensic Sciences* 57, no. 2 (March 2012): 398–412. https://doi.org/10.1111/j.1556-4029.2011.02008.x.

Amazon Conservation Team. *The Amazonian Travels of Richard Evans Schultes* (storymap) (2018). https://www.amazonteam.org/maps/schultes/en/.

Bain, Katie. "Pure Ecstasy." *Playboy* (December 2015). https://www.playboy.com/magazine/articles/2015/12/pure-ecstasy/.

Barker SA. "Administration of N,N-dimethyltryptamine (DMT) in psychedelic therapeutics and research and the study of endogenous DMT." *Psychopharmacology* 239 (2022): 1749–63. https://doi.org/10.1007/s00213-022-06065-0.

Barrett, Frederick S. *The Neuroscience of Psychedelic Drugs, Music, and Nostalgia.* TEDMED Talks (video) (October 1, 2020). https://www.youtube.com/watch?v=sxm8QwvESJk/.

Barrett FS, Robbins H, Smooke D, et al. "Qualitative and quantitative features of music reported to support peak mystical experiences during psychedelic therapy sessions." *Frontiers in Physiology* 8 (July 2017). https://doi.org/10.3389/fpsyg.2017.01238.

Bedi G, Phan KL, Angstadt M, et al. "Effects of MDMA on sociability and neural response to social threat and social reward." *Psychopharmacology* (*Berlin*) 207, no. 1 (November 2009): 73–83. https://doi.org/10.107/s00213-009-1635-z.

Bergman, RL. "Navajo Peyote Use: Its Apparent Safety." *American Journal of Psychiatry* 128, no. 6 (December 1971). https://doi.org /10.1176/ajp.128.6.695.

Bienemann B, Stomato Ruschel N, Campos ML, et al. "Self-reported negative outcomes of psilocybin users: a quantitative textual analysis." *PLoS ONE* 15, no. 2 (February 21, 2020): e0229067. https://doi.org/10.1371 /journal.pone.0229067.

BioSpace, "Small Pharma Reports Positive Top-line Results from Phase IIa Trial of SPL026 in Major Depressive Disorder" (January 25, 2023). https://www.biospace.com/small -pharma-reports-positive-top-line-results -from-phase-iia-trial-of-spl026-in-major -depressive-disorder.

Bogenschutz MP, Ross S, Bhatt S, et al. "Percentage of heavy drinking days following psilocybin-assisted psycho-therapy vs placebo in the treatment of adult patients with alcohol use disorder: a randomized clinical trial." *JAMA Psychiatry* 79, no. 10 (2022): 953–62. https://doi .org/10.1001/jamapsychiatry.2022.2096.

Bourzat, Francine. *Consciousness Medicine: Indigenous Wisdom, Entheogens, and Expanded States of Consciousness for Healing and Growth.* North Atlantic Books, 2019.

Bouso JC, González D, Fondevila S, et al. "Personality, psychopathology, life attitudes and neuropsychological performance among ritual users of ayahuasca: a longitudinal study." *PLoS ONE* 7, no. 8 (August 8, 2012): e42421. https://doi.org /10.1371/journal.pone.0042421.

Boyle NT, Connor TJ. "Methylenedioxymethamphetamine ('Ecstasy')-induced immunosuppression: a cause for concern?" *British Journal of Pharmacology* 161, no. 1 (September 2010): 17–32. https://doi.org/10.1111/j.1476 -5381.2010.00899.x.

Brasher, Trey. "The overlapping history of beta-blockers and psilocybin." *Unlimited Sciences* (blog). (July 7, 2022). https:// unlimitedsciences.org/the-overlapping -history-of-beta-blockers-and-psilocybin/.

Breen, Benjamin. "How Margaret Mead's Research into Utopias Helped Usher in the Psychedelic Era." Interview by Terry Gross. NPR: *Fresh Air* (January 16, 2024). https:// www.npr.org/2024/01/16/1224894129 /margaret-meads-psychedelics-benjamin -breen-tripping-on-utopia.

Brown TK, Alper K. "Treatment of opioid use disorder with ibogaine: detoxification and drug use outcomes." *American Journal of Drug and Alcohol Abuse* 44, no. 1 (2018): 24–36. https://doi.org/10.1080/00952990.20 17.1320802.

Browne, Grace. "Psychedelic therapy is here. Just don't call it therapy." *Wired* (June 15, 2023). https://www.wired.com/story/oregon -psychedelics-psilocybin-rollout/.

Cable, Josh. "Study: Ibogaine Shows Promise in Treating Symptoms of Traumatic Brain Injury in Veterans." *Psychedelic Medical News* (January 16, 2024). https://psychedelic medicalnews.com/ibogaine-shows-promise -treating-symptoms-traumatic-braininjury/.

Calder AE, Hasler G. "Towards an understanding of psychedelic-induced neuroplasticity." *Neuropsychopharmacology* 48 (2023): 104–12. https://www.nature.com/articles /s41386-022-01389-z.

Carhart-Harris RL, Bolstridge M, Rucker J, et al. "Psilocybin with psychological support for treatment-resistant depression: an open-label feasibility study." *Lancet Psychiatry* 3, no. 7 (July 2016): 619–27. https://doi.org /10.1016/S2215-0366(16)30065-7.

Carhart-Harris RL, Erritzoe D, Williams T, et al. "Neural correlates of the entheogen state as determined by fMRI studies with psilocybin." *Proceedings of the National Academy of Sciences* 109, no. 6 (February 2012): https://doi.org/10.1073/pnas.1119598109.

Carhart-Harris RL, Friston KJ. "REBUS and the anarchic brain: toward a unified model of the brain action of psychedelics." *Pharmacological Reviews* 7, no. 13 (July 2019): 316–44. https://doi.org/10.1124/pr.118017160.

Carhart-Harris RL, Kaelen M, Nutt DJ. "How do hallucinogens work on the brain?" *Psychologist* (2014): 662–65.

Carhart-Harris RL, Leech R, Hellyer PJ, et al. "The entropic brain: a theory of conscious states informed by neuroimaging research with psychedelic drugs." *Frontiers in Human Neuroscience* 8 (February 2, 2012). https://doi.org/10.3389/fnhum.2014.00020.

Callaway J. "Ayahuasca Preparations and Serotonin Reuptake Inhibitors: A Potential Combination for Severe Adverse Interactions." *Journal of Psychoactive Drugs* 30, no. 9 (1998): pp. 367–69. https://www.researchgate.net/publication/13364059_Ayahuasca_Preparations_and_Serotonin_Reuptake_Inhibitors_A_Potential_Combination_for_Severe_Adverse Interactions.

Canadian Institutes of Health Research. "Psilocybin-Assisted Psychotherapy Research Grant." (June 29, 2023). https://www.canada.ca/en/institutes-health-research/news/2023/06/psilocybin-assisted-psychotherapy-research-grant.html/.

Cavanna F, Muller S, de la Fuente LA, et al. "Microdosing with psilocybin mushrooms: a double-blind placebo-controlled study." *Translational Psychiatry* 12, no. 307 (2022). https://doi.org/10.1038/s41398-022-02039-0.

Cherian KN, Keynan JN, Anker L, et al. "Magnesium–ibogaine therapy in veterans with traumatic brain injuries." *Nature Medicine* 30 (2024): 373–81. https://doi.org/10.1038/s41591-023-02705-w.

Christie D, Yazar-Klosinski B, Nosova E, et al. "MDMA-assisted therapy is associated with a reduction in chronic pain among people with post-traumatic stress disorder." *Frontiers in Psychiatry* 13 (November 2, 2022). https://doi.org/10.3389/fpsyt.2022.939302.

Cohen, Stefanie. "Inside the 1950s LSD Therapy That Changed Cary Grant's Life." *Vulture* (June 22, 2017). https://www.vulture.com/2017/06/cary-grants-lsd-therapy-the-inside-story.html.

Daley P, McCombs D, Ogunbodede O, Terry M, et al. "New Mescaline Concentrations from 14 Taxa/Cultivars of Echinopsis spp. (Cactaceae) ('San Pedro') and Their Relevance to Shamanic Practice," *Journal of Ethnopharmacology* 131, no. 2 (2010): Issue 2, 356–362. https://www.sciencedirect.com/science/article/abs/pii/S0378874110004836?via%3Dihub.

Danforth AL, Grob CS, Struble C, et al. "Reduction in social anxiety after MDMA-assisted psychotherapy with autistic adults: a randomized, double-blind, placebo-controlled pilot study." *Psychopharmacology* 235, no. 11 (September 2018): 3137–48. https://doi.org/10.1007/s00213-018-5010-9.

Dasgupta, Amitava. "Abuse of Magic Mushroom, Peyote Cactus, LSD, and Volatiles." In

*Critical Issues in Alcohol and Drugs Abuse Testing*, edited by Amitava Dasgupta. Academic Press, 2019. https://doi.org/10.1016/B978-0-12-815607-0.00033-2.

Das, Rameshawar. *Being Ram Dass*. Sounds True, 2021. CD-ROM.

Davis AK, Averill LA, Sepeda ND, et al. "Psychedelic treatment for trauma-related psychological and cognitive impairment among US special operations forces veterans." *Chronic Stress* 4 (July 8, 2020). https://doi.org/10.1177/2470547020939564.

Davis AK, So S, Lancelotta R, et al. "5-methoxy-N,N-dimethyltryptamine (5-MeO-DMT) used in a naturalistic group setting is associated with unintended improvements in depression and anxiety." *American Journal of Drug and Alcohol Abuse* 45, no. 2 (2019): 161–69. https://doi.org/10.1080/00952990.2018.1545024.

Davis, Erik. *Blotter: The Untold Story of an Acid Medium*. MIT Press, 2024.

Davis W, Weil AT. "Identity of a new world psychoactive toad." *Ancient Mesoamerica* 3, no. 1 (1992): 51–59. https://doi.org/10.1017/S0956536100002297.

de Loenen, Ben (dir.). *Ibogaine: Rite of Passage*. LunArt Productions, ICEERS (video) (2004). https://www.youtube.com/watch?v=vt0E8N4FRFY/.

DeRienzo, Paul. "The Ibogaine Alternative." *Cannabis Culture* (November 29, 2005). https://www.cannabisculture.com/content/2005/11/29/4584/.

Dickinson, Jonathan. "Could Ibogaine Be a Promising New Treatment for Parkinson's Disease?" *Ambio* (blog), December 20, 2022. https://ambio.life/blog/could-ibogaine-be-a-promising-new-treatment-for-parkinsons-disease/.

Doblin R. "Pahnke's 'Good Friday Experiment': a long-term follow-up and methodological critique." *Journal of Transpersonal Psychology* 23, no. 1 (1991): 1–28. https://maps.org/research-archive/cluster/psilo-lsd/goodfriday.pdf.

Doblin R. "Dr. Leary's Concord prison experiment: a 34-year follow-up study." *Journal of Psychoactive Drugs* 30, no. 4 (1998): 419–26. https://doi.org/10.1080/02791072.1998.10399715.

Doblin, Rick. "Rick Doblin." Interview with Joe Rogan (host). *The Joe Rogan Experience* 1661 (podcast) (June 4, 2021). https://maps.org/2021/06/04/the-joe-rogan-experience-1661-rick-doblin/.

Dolce, Joe. *Brave New Weed: Adventures into the Uncharted World of Cannabis*. Harper Wave, 2016.

Dubley, Phil. "Interactions Between Kratom & Magic Mushrooms." n.d. https://kratom.org/interactions/magic-mushrooms/.

Dumont GJH, Sweep FCGJ, van der Steen R, et al. "Increased oxytocin concentrations and prosocial feelings in humans after ecstasy (3,4-methylenedioxymethamphetamine) administration." *Social Neuroscience* 4, no. 4 (2009): 359–66. https://doi.org/10.1080/17470910802649470.

Dyck, Erika. *Psychedelics: A Visual Odyssey*. MIT Press, 2024.

Edakubo S, Fushimi K. "Mortality and risk assessment for anorexia nervosa in acute-care hospitals: a nationwide administrative database analysis." *BMC Psychiatry* 20, no. 1 (January 13, 2020): 19. https://doi.org/10.1186/s12888-020-2433-8.

Edsinger E, Dölen G. "A conserved role for serotonergic neurotransmission in mediating social behavior in octopus."

*Current Biology* 28, no. 19 (October 2018): 3136–42. https://doi.org/10.1016/j.cub.2018.07.061.

Evans, Jules. "Unveiling the Shadows: Jules Evans on Challenging Psychedelic Experiences." *Mind Body Health & Politics* (podcast) (March 5, 2024). https://lnns.co/DxgAL_aBv2w.

Eisner, Bruce. *Ecstasy: The MDMA Story.* Ronin Publishing, 1989.

Ezquerra-Romano I, Lawn W, Krupitsky E, et al. "Ketamine for the treatment of addiction: evidence and potential mechanisms." *Neuropharmacology* 142 (2018): 72–82. https://doi.org/10.1016/j.neuropharm.2018.01.017.

Fadiman, James. "Psychedelics and the Self: A Conversation with James Fadiman." Interview with Sam Harris (host). *Making Sense* 242 (podcast) (March 23, 2021). https://www.samharris.org/podcasts/making-sense-episodes/242-psychedelics-self.

Fadiman, James. "The Remarkable Results of Microdosing." Science and Nonduality (SAND) Conference 2018 (video) (April 18, 2019). https://www.youtube.com/watch?v=6AfFM8pfy4s.

Favaron, Pedro, and Marcio Pérez (dir.). Explicación de los cantos medicinales Ikaros (video) (March 18, 2019). https://www.youtube.com/watch?v=r5P1RqUkzws.

Fadiman, James. *The Psychedelic Explorer's Guide: Safe, Therapeutic, and Sacred Journeys.* Park Street Press, 2011.

Ferriss, Tim. "Psychedelics—Microdosing, Mind-Enhancing Methods, and More." *The Tim Ferriss Show* 377 (podcast) (July 17, 2019). https://tim.blog/2019/07/17/the-tim-ferriss-show-transcripts-psychedelics-microdosing-mind-enhancing-methods-and-more-377/.

Gandy S, Bonnelle V, Jacobs E, et al. "Psychedelics as potential catalysts of scientific creativity and insight." *Drug Science, Policy and Law* 8 (May 16, 2002). https://doi org/10.1177/20503245221097649.

Gasperi V, Sibilano M, Savini I, et al. "Niacin in the central nervous system: an update of biological aspects and clinical applications." *International Journal of Molecular Sciences* 20, no. 4 (February 23, 2019): 974. https://doi.org/10.3390/ijms20040974.

Gerber K, García Flores I, Ruiz AC, et al. "Ethical concerns about psilocybin intellectual property." *ACS Pharmacology and Translational Science* 4, no. 2 (2021): 573–77. https://doi.org/10.1021/acsptsci.0c00171.

Golden, Hallie. "Inside the Battle to Save the Sacred Peyote Ceremony: 'We're in Dire Straits.'" *Guardian* (December 9, 2022). https://www.theguardian.com/us-news/2022/dec/09/peyote-native-american-medicine-nacna-federal-protection.

Griffiths RR, Hurwitz ES, Davis AK, et al. "Survey of subjective 'God encounter experiences': Comparisons among naturally occurring experiences and those occasioned by the classic psychedelics psilocybin, LSD, ayahuasca, or DMT." *PLoS ONE* 14, no. 4 (2019): e0213377. https://doi.org/10.1371/journal.pone.0214377.

Griffiths RR, Johnson MW, Carducci MA, et al. "Psilocybin produces substantial and sustained decreases in depression and anxiety in patients with life-threatening cancer: a randomized double-blind trial." *Journal of Psychopharmacology* 30, no. 12 (2016): 1181–97. http://doi.org/10.1177/0269881116675513.

Griffiths RR, Richards WA, McCann U, et al. "Psilocybin can occasion mystical-type experiences having substantial and sustained personal meaning and spiritual significance." *Psychopharmacology* 187 (2006): 268–83. https://doi.org/ 10.1007 /s00213-006-0457-5.

Grinspoon L, Doblin R. "Psychedelics as catalysts of insight-oriented psychotherapy." *Social Research* 68, no. 3 (2001): 677–95. http://www.jstor.org/stable/40971906.

Grob CS, McKenna DJ, Callaway JC, et al. "Human psychopharmacology of hoasca, a plant hallucinogen used in ritual context in Brazil." *Journal of Nervous and Mental Disease* 184, no. 2 (February 1996): 86–94. https://doi.org/10.1097/00005053 -199602000-00004.

Grob, Charles (ed). *Hallucinogens: A Reader.* Jeremy Tarcher/Putnam, 2002.

Gukasyan N, Davis AK, Barrett FS, et al. "Efficacy and safety of psilocybin-assisted treatment for major depressive disorder: prospective 12-month follow-up." *Journal of Psychopharmacology* 36, no. 2 (2022): 151–58. https://doi. org/10.1177/02698811211073759.

Hachumak, with David L. Carroll. *Journeying Through the Invisible: The Craft of Healing with, and Beyond, Sacred Plants, as Told by a Peruvian Medicine Man.* Harper, 2022.

Haijen ECHM, Hurks PPM, Kuypers KPC. "Effects of psychedelic microdosing versus conventional ADHD medication use on emotion regulation, empathy, and ADHD symptoms in adults with severe ADHD symptoms: a naturalistic prospective comparison study." *European Psychiatry* 67, no. 1 (2024): e18. https://doi.org/10.1192/j .eurpsy.2024.8.

Halpern JH, Sherwood AR, Hudson JI, et al. "Psychological and cognitive effects of long-term peyote use among Native Americans." *Biological Psychiatry* 58, no. 8 (October 15, 2005): 624–31. https://doi.org/10.1016/j .biopsych.2005.06.038.

Halpern JH, Sherwood AR, Hudson JI, et al. "Residual neurocognitive features of long-term ecstasy users with minimal exposure to other drugs." *Addiction* 106, no. 4 (April 2011): 777–86. https://doi.org/10.1111/j.1360 -0443.2010.03252.x.

Hanna J, Thyssen S. "Talking with Ann and Sasha Shulgin: on the existence of God and the pleasure of sex drugs." *MAPS Journal: Sex, Spirit and Psychedelics* 12, no.1 (2002): 3–6. https://maps.org/news-letters/v12n1 /12103shu.pdf.

Harris, Rachel. *Listening to Ayahuasca: New Hope for Depression, Addiction, PTSD, and Anxiety.* New World Library, 2017.

Harris, Rachel. *Swimming in the Sacred: Wisdom from the Psychedelic Underground.* New World Library, 2023.

Hartogsohn, Ido. *American Trip: Set, Setting, and the Psychedelic Experience in the Twentieth Century.* MIT Press, 2020.

Heaven, Ross. *Cactus of Mystery: The Shamanic Powers of the Peruvian San Pedro Cactus.* Park Street Press, 2013.

Hofmann, Albert. *LSD: My Problem Child: Reflections on Sacred Drugs, Mysticism and Science.* Multidisciplinary Association for Psychedelic Studies (MAPS), 1979.

Hofmann, Albert. "*High Times* Greats: Interview with Albert Hofmann, the Man Who First Synthesized LSD." *High Times* (July 1976). https://hightimes.com/culture/albert -hofmann-lsd-interview/.

Hofmann, Albert, and Richard Evans Schultes. *Plants of the Gods: Origins of Hallucinogenic Use*. McGraw-Hill, 1979.

Holland, Julie (ed). *Ecstasy: The Complete Guide: A Comprehensive Look at the Risks and Benefits of MDMA*. Park Street Press, 2001.

Holland, Julie. *Good Chemistry: The Science of Connection, from Soul to Psychedelics*. Harper, 2020.

Holler JM, Vorce SP, McDonough-Bender PC, et al. "A drug toxicity death involving propylhexedrine and mitragynine." *Journal of Analytical Toxicology* 35, no 1 (January 2011): 54–59. https://doi.org/10.1093/anatox/35.1.54.

Hu, Jane C. "Ketamine's Abuse Potential: Five Questions for Psychiatrist Jennifer Swainson." The Microdose (September 30, 2024). https://themicrodose.substack.com/p/ketamines-abuse-potential-5-questions.

Huberman, Andrew. "The Science of MDMA & Its Therapeutic Uses: Benefits & Risks." Huberman Lab Podcast (podcast video) (June 12, 2023) https://www.youtube.com/watch?v=slUCmZJDXrk.

Hull TD, Malgaroli M, Gazzaley A, et al. "At-home, sublingual ketamine telehealth is a safe and effective treatment for moderate to severe anxiety and depression: findings from a large, prospective, open-label effectiveness trial." *Journal of Affective Disorders* 314 (October 1, 2022): 59–67. https://doi.org/10.1016/j.jad.2022.07.004.

Huxley, Aldous. *The Doors of Perception*. Harper & Row, 1954.

Institute for Quality and Efficiency in Health Care (IQWiG). "How Effective Are Anti-depressants?" (updated 2024). https://www.ncbi.nlm.nih.gov/books/NBK361016.

Jay, Mike. *Mescaline: A Global History of the First Psychedelic*. Yale University Press, 2019.

Jay, Mike. "What Happened to Mescaline?" Yale University Press Catalog, August 6, 2019. https://yalebooks.yale.edu/2019/08/06/what-happened-to-mescaline/.

Johnson, Matthew W. "The Ultimate Psychedelics Explainer" *The Big Think Interview* (video) (n.d.). https://bigthink.com/series/the-big-think-interview/ultimate-psychedelics-explainer/.

Johnson MW, Garcia-Romeu A, Cosimano MP, et al. "Pilot study of the 5-HT$_{2A}$R agonist psilocybin in the treatment of tobacco addiction." *Journal of Psychopharmacology* 28, no 11 (September 2014): 983–992. https://doi.org/10.1177/0269881114548296.

Johnson MW, Garcia-Romeu A, Griffiths RR. "Long-term follow-up of psilocybin-facilitated smoking cessation." *American Journal of Drug and Alcohol Abuse* 43, no. 1 (2016): 55–60. https://doi.org/10.3109/00952990.2016.1170135.

Johnson MW, Richards WA, Griffiths RR. "Human hallucinogen research: guidelines for safety." *Journal of Psychopharmacology* 22, no. 6 (August 2008): 603–20. https://doi.org/10.1177/0269881108093587.

Joshi, Shamani. "Love and other drugs: the couples using psychedelics as a way to get closer." Vice.com (February 28, 2022). https://www.vice.com/en/article/bvnpjq/couples-doing-psychedelic-drugs-lsd-mushrooms-therapy-relationship-sex.

Karst M, Halpern JH, Bernateck M, et al. "The non-hallucinogen 2-bromo-lysergic acid diethylamide as preventative treatment for cluster headache: an open, non-randomized case series." *Cephalalgia* 30, no. 9 (September 2010): 1140–44.

https://doi.org/10.1177/0333102410363490.

Katchborian-Neto A, Santos MFC, Vilas-Boas DF, et al. "Immunological modulation and control of parasitaemia by ayahuasca compounds: therapeutic potential for Chagas's disease." *Chemistry and Biodiversity* 19, no. 10 (October 2022): e202200409. https://doi.org/10.1002/cbdv.202200409.

Kentucky Attorney General. "Kentucky Opioid Abatement Commission Public Hearing" (video) (July 17, 2023). https://www.youtube.com/watch?v=3-PubzAw6QU.

Kilham, Chris. "Kava, an ethnomedical review" (based on UMass teaching notes, 2000–2005)." Erowid: Plants: Kava (2006). Erowid.org/plants/kava/kava_article1.shtml.

Kinzer, Stephen. "From Mind Control to Murder? How a Deadly Fall Revealed the CIA's Darkest Secrets." *Guardian* (September 6, 2019). https://www.theguardian.com/us-news/2019/sep/06/from-mind-control-to-murder-how-a-deadly-fall-revealed-the-cias-darkest-secrets.

"Kratom." National Institute on Drug Abuse (March 25, 2022). https://nida.nih.gov/research-topics/kratom.

Krebs TS, Johansen PO. "Over 30 million psychedelic users in the United States." *F1000Research* 2, no. 98 (2013). https://doi.org/10.12688/f1000research.2-98.v1.

Lai PL, Naidu M, Sabaratnam V, et al. "Neurotrophic properties of the lion's mane medicinal mushroom, *Hericium erinaceus* (higher basidiomycetes) from Malaysia." *International Journal of Medicinal Mushrooms* 15, no. 6 (2013): 539–54. https://doi.org/10.1615/intjmedmushr.v15.i6.30.

Langlitz, Nicolas. *Neuropsychedelia: The Revival of Hallucinogenic Research since the Decade of the Brain.* University of California Press, 2012.

Lattin, Don. *Distilled Spirits: Getting High, Then Sober, with a Famous Writer, a Forgotten Philosopher, and a Hopeless Drunk.* University of California Press, 2012.

Lett S. "Psychedelics and music: listening for liberation." *MAPS Bulletin* 34, no. 1 (April 12, 2024). https://maps.org/news/bulletin/psychedelic-music-listening-liberation/.

*LSD in the United States* (report). US Drug Enforcement Administration, Strategic Intelligence Section, Domestic Unit, 1995.

Ma BJ, Shen JW, et al. "Hericenones and erinacines: stimulators of nerve growth factor (NGF) biosynthesis in *Hericium erinaceus.*" *Mycology* 1, no. 2 (2010): 92–98. https://doi.org/10.1080/21501201003735556.

Manganyi MC, Bezuidenhout CC, Regnier T, et al. "A chewable cure 'kanna': biological and pharmaceutical properties of *Sceletium tortuosum.*" *Molecules* 26, no. 9 (April 28, 2021): 2557. https://doi.org/10.3390/molecules26092557.

Markoff, John. *What the Doormouse Said: How the Sixties Counterculture Shaped the Personal Computer Industry.* Penguin Books, 2006.

Mash, Deborah. "MINDSET Lecture Series: Deborah Mash, PhD." Icahn School of Medicine (video) (January 12, 2022). https://www.youtube.com/watch?v=Drtk2SQM_gI.

Mash DC. "IUPHAR—invited review—ibogaine—a legacy within the current renaissance of psychedelic therapy." *Pharmacological Research* 190 (April 2023): 106620. https://doi.org/10.1016/j.phrs.2022.106620.

McConnell, Patrick. "A beginner's guide to San Pedro." *Double Blind* (May 2, 2024). https://doubleblindmag.com/san-pedro/.

McKenna, Dennis J. "The healing vine: ayahuasca as medicine in the 21st century." In Winkelman, Michael J., and Thomas B. Roberts (eds.), *Psychedelic Medicine: New Evidence for Hallucinogenic Substances as Treatments*, vol. 1. Praeger Publishers, 2007, 21–44.

McKenna, Dennis. *Brotherhood of the Screaming Abyss: My Life with Terence McKenna.* Synergetic Press, 2012.

McKenna, Terence. *Food of the Gods: The Search for the Original Tree of Knowledge: A Radical History of Plants, Drugs, and Human Evolution.* Bantam, 1992.

McNeil Jr., Donald G. "Research on Ecstasy Is Clouded by Errors." *New York Times* (December 2, 2003). https://www.nytimes.com/2003/12/02/science/research-on-ecstasy-is-clouded-by-errors.html.

Merabet LB, Maguire D, Warde A, et al. "Visual hallucinations during prolonged blindfolding in sighted subjects." *Journal of Neuro-Opthalmology* 24, no. 2 (June 2004): 109–13. https://doi.org/10.1097/00041327-200406000-00003.

Metzner, Ralph (ed). *The Ayahuasca Experience: A Sourcebook on the Sacred Vine of Spirits.* Park Street Press, 1999.

"MindMed Receives FDA Breakthrough Therapy Designation and Announces Positive 12-Week Durability Data From Phase 2B Study of MM120 for Generalized Anxiety Disorder." BusinessWire (press release) (March 7, 2024). https://www.businesswire.com/news/home/20240307733599/en/.

Mithoefer MC, Wagner MT, Mithoefer AT, et al. " The safety and efficacy of ±3,4-methylenedioxymethamphetamine-assisted psychotherapy in subjects with chronic, treatment-resistant posttraumatic stress disorder: the first randomized controlled pilot study." *Journal of Psychopharmacology* 25, no. 4 (2011): 439–52. https://doi.org/10.1177/0269881110378371.

Molla H, Lee R, Tare I, et al. "Greater subjective effects of a low dose of LSD in participants with depressed mood." *Neuropsychopharmacology* 49 (2024): 774–81. https://doi.org/10.1038/s41386-023-01772-4.

Morales-García JA, de la Fuente Revenga M, Alonso-Gil S, et al. "The alkaloids of *Banisteriopsis caapi*, the plant source of the Amazonian hallucinogen ayahuasca, stimulate adult neurogenesis in vitro." *Scientific Reports* 7, no. 5309 (2017). https://doi.org/10.1038/s41598-017-05407-9.

Morris, Hamilton A., and Ash Smith. "The Last Interview with Alexander Shulgin." Vice.com (video) (May 1, 2010). https://www.vice.com/en/article/the-last-interview-with-alexander-shulgin-423-v17n5/.

Morris, Hamilton A., and Ash Smith. "SiHKL: Shulgins I Have Known and Loved." Vice.com (December 22, 2010). https://www.vice.com/en/article/sihkal-shulgins-i-have-known-and-loved/.

Muraresku, Brian C. "Natural Born Visionaries." *Field Tripping* (podcast). https://www.youtube.com/watch?v=HTLBeROoHzY.

Multidisciplinary Association for Psychedelic Studies (MAPS). "FDA Grants Breakthrough Therapy Designation for MDMA-Assisted Therapy for PTSD" (August 26, 2017). https://maps.org/news/media/press-release-fda-grants-breakthrough-therapy

-designation-for-mdma-assisted
-psychotherapy-for-ptsd-agrees-on
-special-protocol-assessment-for-phase
-3-trials/.

Narby, Jeremy. *The Cosmic Serpent: DNA and the Origins of Knowledge.* Jeremy Tarcher/Putnam, 1998.

Narby, Jeremy, and Rafael Chanchari Pizuri. *Plant Teachers: Ayahuasca, Tobacco, and the Pursuit of Knowledge.* New World Library, 2021.

Nardou R, Lewis EM, Rothhaas R, et al. "Oxytocin-dependent reopening of a social reward learning critical period with MDMA." *Nature* 569 (2019): 116–20. https://doi.org/10.1038/s41586-019-1075-9.

Nardou R, Sawyer E, Song YJ, et al. "Psychedelics reopen the social reward learning critical period." *Nature* 618 (2023): 790–98. https://doi.org/10.1038/s41586-023-06204-3/.

National Alliance on Mental Illness (NAMI). "Mental Health by the Numbers" (n.d.). https://www.nami.org/about-mental-illness/mental-health-by-the numbers/#/.

Neumann J, Azatsian, K, Höhm C. et al. "Cardiac effects of ephedrine, norephedrine, mescaline, and 3, 4-methylenedioxymethamphetamine (MDMA) in mouse and human atrial preparations." Naunyn-Schmiedeberg's Archives of Pharmacology 396 (2023): 275–87. https://doi.org/10.1007/s00210-022-02315-2.

Nicholas CR, Wang JG, Coker A, et al. "The effects of MDMA-assisted therapy on alcohol and substance use in a phase 3 trial for treatment of severe PTSD." *Drug and Alcohol Dependence* 233 (April 1, 2022). https://doi.org/10.1016/j.drugalcdep.2022.109356.

Nichols DE. "N,N-dimethyltryptamine and the pineal gland: separating fact from myth." *Journal of Psychopharmacology* 32, no. 1 (2018): 30–36. https://doi.org/10.1177/0269881117736919.

Noller GE, Frampton CM, Yazar-Klosinski B. "Ibogaine treatment outcomes for opioid dependence from a twelve-month follow-up observational study." *American Journal of Drug and Alcohol Abuse* 44, no. 1 (2018): 37–46. https://doi.org/10.1080/00952990.2017.1310218.

Nutt, David. *Psychedelics: The Revolutionary Drugs That Could Change Your Life—A Guide from the Expert.* Hachette Books, 2024.

Nuwer, Rachel. "How MDMA Became the Club Drug of the Century." *Daily Beast* (June 3, 2023). https://www.thedailybeast.com/how-mdma-became-the-club-drug-of-the-century/.

Nuwer, Rachel. "Understanding MDMA." Interview with Danielle Venton. Commonwealth Club (June 15, 2023). https://www.commonwealthclub.org/events/archive/podcast/rachel-nuwer-understanding-mdma.

Nuwer, Rachel. *MDMA and the Quest for Connection in a Fractured World.* Bloomsbury Publishing, 2023.

Ogunbodede O, McCombs D, Trout K, et al. "New mescaline concentrations from 14 taxa/cultivars of Echinopsis spp. (Cactaceae) ('San Pedro') and their relevance to shamanic practice." *Journal of Ethnopharmacology* 131, no. 2 (2010): 356–62. https://doi.org/10.1016/j.jep.2010.07.021.

Ohler, Norman. *Tripped: Nazi Germany, the CIA, and the Dawn of the Psychedelic Age.* Mariner Books, 2024.

Olson, David. "Does Psychedelic Therapy Need the Trip?" Interview with Steve Paulson. *To the Best of Our Knowledge* (podcast) (December 16, 2023). https://www.ttbook.org/interview/does-psychedelic-therapy-need-trip/.

"One Pill Can Kill: DEA Fentanyl Seizures in 2024." US Drug Enforcement Administration (n.d.). dea.gov/onepill.

Orhurhu VJ, Vashisht R, Claus LE, et al. "Ketamine Toxicity." *StatPearls* (2024). https://www.ncbi.nlm.nih.gov/books/NBK541087/

Ortiz Bernal AM, Raison CL, Lancelotta RL, et al. "Reactivations after 5-methoxy-N,N-dimethyltryptamine use in naturalistic settings: an initial exploratory analysis of the phenomenon's predictors and its emotional valence." *Frontiers in Psychiatry* 13 (November 29, 2022). https://doi.org/10.3389/fpsyt.2022.1049643.

Oss O. T., O. N. Oeric, and Terence McKenna. *Psilocybin: Magic Mushroom Grower's Guide: A Handbook for Psilocybin Enthusiasts.* QuickAmerican Publishing, 1976.

Page, Ben. *Healing Trees: A Pocket Guide to Forest Bathing.* Mandala Publishing, n.d.

Park, Ashley. "Psychedelic Drugs and the Fine Arts in the 1960s and 1970s." *Ibid.: A Student History Journal*, vol 12. Texas Woman's University, 2019. https://twu.edu/media/documents/history-government/Psychedelic-Drugs-and-the-Fine-Arts-in-the-1960-and-1970.pdf.

Passie T. "The early use of MDMA ('Ecstasy') in psychotherapy (1977–1985)." *Drug Science, Policy and Law* 4 (2018). https://doi.org/10.1177/2050324518767442.

Passie, Torsten. *The History of MDMA.* Oxford University Press, 2023.

Pellerin, Cheryl. *Trips: How Hallucinogens Work in Your Brain.* Seven Stories Press, 1998.

Peugh J, Belenko S. "Alcohol, drugs, and sexual function: a review." *Journal of Psychoactive Drugs* 33, no. 3 (July–September 2001): https://doi.org/10.1080/02791072.2001.10400569.

Pickard, William Leonard. *The Rose of Paracelsus: On Secrets & Sacraments.* Synergetic Press, 2023.

Pinchbeck, Daniel. "Ten Years of Therapy in One Night." *Guardian* (September 19, 2003). https://www.theguardian.com/books/2003/sep/20/booksonhealth.lifeandhealth.

Plotkin, Mark J., host, *Plants of the Gods: Hallucinogens, Healing, Culture and Conservation* podcast, season 6, episode 7, "Medicinal Plants and the Fungi of the Amazon," October 2, 2024, https://podcasts.apple.com/us/podcast/plants-of-the-gods-s6e7-the-medicinal/id1549464922?i=1000671515213.

Plotkin, Mark J. *Tales of a Shaman's Apprentice: An Ethnobotanist Searches for New Medicines in the Rain Forest.* Penguin Books, 1993.

Pollan, Michael. *How to Change Your Mind: What the New Science of Psychedelics Teaches Us About Consciousness, Dying, Addiction, Depression, and Transcendence.* Penguin Press, 2018.

Preller KH, Razi A, Zeidman P, et al. "Effective connectivity changes in LSD-induced altered states of consciousness in humans." *Proceedings of the National Academy of Sciences* 116, no. 7 (2019): 2743–48. https://doi.org/10.1073/pnas.1815129116.

Price R. "Looking at smiling faces extends the antidepressant effects of ketamine." *PittWire* 28 (September 2022).

Price R, Spotts C, Panny B, et al. "A Novel, Brief, Fully Automated Intervention to Extend the Antidepressant Effect of a Single Ketamine Infusion: A Randomized Clinical Trial." *American Journal of Psychiatry* 179, no. 12 (September 2022). https://doi.org/10.1176/appi.ajp.20220216.

Qing, Li. *Forest Bathing: How Trees Can Help You Find Health and Happiness.* Penguin Life, 2018.

Ramaekers JG, Hutten N, Mason NL, et al. "A low dose of lysergic acid diethylamide decreases pain perception in healthy volunteers." *Journal of Psychopharmacology* 35, no. 4 (2021): 398–405. https://doi.org/10.1177/0269881120940937.

Reckweg JT, van Leeuwen CJ, Henquet C, et al. "A phase 1/2 trial to assess safety and efficacy of a vaporized 5-methoxy-N,N-dimethyltryptamine formulation (GH001) in patients with treatment-resistant depression." *Frontiers in Psychiatry* 14 (June 20, 2023). https://doi.org/10.3389/fpsyt.2023.1133414.

Rees, Alun. "Nobel Prize genius Crick was high on LSD when he discovered the secret of life, https://maps.org/2004/08/08/nobel-prize-genius-crick-was-high-on-lsd-when-he-discovered-dna/." *Mail on Sunday* (August 8, 2004).

Reneman L, Lavalaye J, Schmand B, et al. "Cortical serotonin transporter density and verbal memory in individuals who stopped using 3,4-methylenedioxymethamphetamine (MDMA or 'Ecstasy'): preliminary findings." *Archives of General Psychiatry* 58, no. 10 (2001): 901–06. https://doi.org/10.1001/archpsyc.58.10.901.

Rich, Ryan. "Iboga and ibogaine harm reduction." *Psychedelic Support* (blog) (June 15, 2021). https://psychedelic.support/resources/iboga-ibogaine-harm-reduction/.

Rootman JM, Kiraga M, Kryskow P, et al. "Psilocybin microdosers demonstrate greater observed improvements in mood and mental health at one month relative to non-microdosing controls." *Scientific Reports* 12, no. 11091 (2022). https://doi.org/10.1038/s41598-022-14512-3.

Rosenbaum SB, Gupta V, Patel P, et al. "Ketamine [updated January 30, 2024]." *StatPearls* (2024). https://www.ncbi.nlm.nih.gov/books/NBK470357/.

Rosin, Hanna. "You Won't Feel High After Watching This Video." *The Cut* (March 22, 2022). https://www.thecut.com/2022/03/you-wont-feel-high-after-watching-this-video.html.

Ross S, Bossis A, Guss J, et al. "Rapid and sustained symptom reduction following psilocybin treatment for anxiety and depression in patients with life-threatening cancer: a randomized controlled trial." *Journal of Psychopharmacology* 30, no.12 (2016): 1165–80. https://doi.org/10.1177/0269881116675512.

Ruffell SGD, Crosland-Wood M, Palmer R, et al. "Ayahuasca: a review of historical, pharmacological, and therapeutic aspects." *Psychiatry and Clinical Neurosciences Reports* 2, no. 4 (2023): e146. https://doi.org/10.1002/pcn5.146.

Sala, Luc. *Homage to Albert Hofmann 100 Year Basel 2006* (video) (March 4, 2016). https://www.youtube.com/ watch ?v=gHcDDxMaPdw.

Sample, Ian. "Psychedelic Brew Ayahuasca's Profound Impact Revealed in Brain Scans." *Guardian* (March 20, 2023). https://www .theguardian.com/science/2023/mar/20 /psychedelic-brew-ayahuasca-profound -impact-brain-scans-dmt.

Schwartzburg, Louie (dir.). *Fantastic Fungi.* Moving Art Studio, 2019.

Schultes, Richard Evans. "The appeal of peyote (*Lophophora williamsii*) as a medicine." *American Anthropologist* (October– December 1938): 698–715.

Schultes, Richard Evans. *Peyote and Plants Used in the Peyote Ceremony.* Botanical Museum Leaflets, Harvard University (1937).

Schultes, Richard Evans, Albert Hofmann, and Christian Ratsch. *Plants of the Gods: Their Sacred, Healing and Hallucinogenic Powers.* Healing Arts Press, 1998.

Sessa B. "The history of psychedelics in medicine." In M. von Heyden, H. Jungaberle, and T. Majić (eds.), *Handbuch Psychoaktive Substanzen.* Springer Reference Psychologie. Springer, 2016. https://doi.org/10.1007/978-3 -642-55214-4_96-1.

Sessa B, Sakal C, O'Brien S, et al. "First study of safety and tolerability of 3,4-methylenedioxymethamphetamine (MDMA)-assisted psychotherapy in patients with alcohol use disorder: preliminary data on the first four participants." *BMJ Case Reports* 12, no. 7 (July 15, 2019). https://doi.org/10.1136 /bcr-2019-230109.

Sewell RA, Halpern JH, and Pope HG Jr. "Response of cluster headache to psilocybin and LSD." *Neurology* 66, no. 12 (June 27, 2006): 1920–22. https://www.neurology.org /doi/10.1212/01.wnl.0000219761.05466.43

Sherwood AM, Claveau R, Lancelotta R, et al. "Synthesis and Characterization of 5-MeO-DMT Succinate for Clinical Use." *ACS Omega* 5, no. 49 (December 2, 2020). https://doi.org/10.1021/acsomega.0c05099.

Shroder, Tom. "'Apparently Useless': The Accidental Discovery of LSD." *Atlantic* (September 9, 2014). https://www.the atlantic.com/health/archive/2014/09 /the-accidental-discovery-of-lsd/379564.

Shulgin, Alexander, and Ann Shulgin. *PiHKAL: A Chemical Love Story.* Transform Press, 1991.

Shulgin, Alexander, and Ann Shulgin. *TiHKAL: The Continuation.* Transform Press, 1997.

Silman, Anna. "Leave your body at the door: how ketamine became the drug of choice for our dissociated moment." *The Cut* (November 21, 2019). https://www.thecut.com/2019/11 /ketamine-disassociation-generation.html.

Silman, Anna. "Ketamine is being sold as a depression wonder drug. For some, it's making everything worse." *Business Insider* (January 25, 2023). https://www.business insider.com/ketamine-therapy-depression -treatment-addictive-drug-clinics-2023-1.

Singleton SP, Wang JB, Mithoefer M, et al. "Altered brain activity and functional connectivity after MDMA-assisted therapy for post-traumatic stress disorder." *Frontiers in Psychiatry* (January 11, 2023). https://doi.org/10.3389/fpsyt.2022.947622.

Sklerov J, Levine B, Moore KA, et al. "A fatal intoxication following the ingestion of 5-methoxy-N,N-dimethyltryptamine in an ayahuasca preparation." *Journal of Analytical Toxicology* 29, no. 8 (November–December 2005): 838–41. https://doi.org/10.1093/jat/29.8.838.

Small Pharma, Ltd. "SPL026 (DMT Fumarate) in Healthy Subjects and MDD Patients" (report) (March 27, 2024). https://www.clinicaltrials.gov/study/NCT04673383?term=SPL026&rank=1.

Smorin, Anatoli. "Putting more hours in the workday: an experience with kratom." Erowid Experiences: Kratom (August 5, 2021). erowid.org/exp/115535.

Strassman, Rick. *DMT: The Spirit Molecule.* Simon & Schuster, 2012.

Strassman, Rick. *A Practical Guide to Psilocybin, LSD, Ketamine, MDMA, and DMT/Ayahuasca.* Ulysses Press, 2022.

Strassman RJ. "Human psychopharmacology of N,N-dimethyltryptamine." *Behavioural Brain Research* 73, nos. 1–2 (December 15, 1995): 121–24. https://doi.org/10.1016/0166-4328(96)00081-2.

Synthesis Institute. "How to Prepare and Integrate a Psychedelic Experience" (July 2, 2021). https://observatory.synthesisinstitute.com/how-to-prepare-and-integrate-a-psychedelic-experience.

Tiefer L. "Female sexual dysfunction: a case study of disease mongering and activist resistance." *PLoS Medicine* 3, no. 4 (2006): e178. https://doi.org/10.1371/journal.pmed.0030178.

Uthaug MV, Lancelotta R, Van Oorsouw K, et al. "A single inhalation of vapor from dried toad secretion containing 5-methoxy-N,N-dimethyltryptamine (5-MeO-DMT) in a naturalistic setting is related to sustained enhancement of satisfaction with life, mindfulness-related capacities, and a decrement of psychopathological symptoms." *Psychopharmacology* 236, no. 9 (2019): 2653–66. https://doi.org/10.1007/s00213-019-05236-w.

US Drug Enforcement Administration (DEA). "One Pill Can Kill: DEA Fentanyl Seizures in 2024" (n.d.). https://www.dea.gov/onepill.

UNC School of Medicine. "Roth Leads $26.9 Million Project to Create Better Psychiatric Medications" (June 15, 2020). https://news.unchealthcare.org/2020/06/roth-leads-26-9-million-project-to-create-better-psychiatric-medications/.

van der Kolk, Bessel A. "Besel van der Kolk on MDMA-Assisted Therapy for PTSD." Interview with Øystein Nødtvedt (host). *Psykologvirke* 1 (podcast) (August 23, 2021). https://psykologvirke.no/fagstoff/mdma-assisted-therapy-ptsd-bessel-van-der-kolk/.

van der Kolk, Bessel A. *The Body Keeps the Score: Brain, Mind and Body in the Healing of Trauma.* Penguin Books, 2014.

Virdi, Jasmine. "DARPA Funds $27 Million Project to Create Psychedelic-Inspired Psychiatric Drugs Without the Trip." *Lucid News* (July 10, 2020). https://www.lucid.news/darpa-funds-project-create-psychedelic-inspired-drugs-without-trip/.

Wagner KD, Fiuty P, Page K, et al. "Prevalence of fentanyl in methamphetamine and cocaine samples collected by community-based drug checking services." *Drug and Alcohol Dependence* 252, no. 110985 (November 1, 2023). https://doi.org/10.1016/j.drugalcdep.2023.110985.

Waldman, Ayalet. *A Really Good Day: How Microdosing Made a Mega Difference in My Mood, My Marriage, and My Life.* Knopf, 2017.

Wallace, AFC. "Cultural Determinants of Response to Hallucinatory Experience." *JAMA Psychiatry* 1, no. 1 (1959): 58–69. https://doi.org/10.1001/archpsyc .1959.03590010074009.

Weil, Andrew. "Dr. Andrew Weil, The New Science of Psychedelics for Mental Health." Interview with Zach Leary (host). *Psychedelics Then and Now with Zach Leary* 38 (podcast) (March 19, 2019). https://maps .org/2019/03/19/maps-podcast-episode-37 -dr-andrew-weil-the-new-science-of -psychedelics-for-mental-health/.

"Weil Says LSD Cured His Allergy." CBS News: *60 Minutes* (March 1, 2001). https://www .cbsnews.com/news/weil-says-lsd-cured -his-allergy-01-03-2001/.

Weiss, Suzannah. "Is Cacao a Psychoactive Substance?" *High Times* (September 29, 2020).

Weiss, Suzannah. "This legal supplement made me roll like I'd taken MDMA." Vice.com (March 9, 2020). https://www.vice.com/en /article/v74xym/kanna-herbal-legal-mdma.

Whitaker-Azmitia PM. "The discovery of serotonin and its role in neuroscience." *Neuropsychopharmacology* 21, Supplement 1 (1999): 2–8. https://doi.org/10.1016/S0893 -133X(99)00031-7.

Winkelman M. "Introduction: evidence for entheogen use in prehistory and world religions." *Journal of Psychedelic Studies* 3, no. 2 (September 13, 2019): 43–62. https:// doi.org/10.1556/2054.2019.024.

Winstock A, Barratt M, Ferris J, et al. *Global Drug Survey 2017* (report) (n.d.). http://www .globaldrugsurvey.com/wp-content/themes /globaldrugsurvey/results/GDS2017_key -findings-report_final.pdf.

Wolfson, Phil, and Glen Hartelius (eds.). *The Ketamine Papers: Science, Therapy, and Transformation.* Multidisciplinary Association for Psychedelic Studies, 2016.

Wright, Webb. "Notes from the Underground Market," *Double Blind*, July 17, 2024, https:// doubleblindmag.com/notes-from-the -underground-mushroom-market/.

Zeifman RJ, Singhal N, Breslow L, et al. "On the relationship between classic psychedelics and suicidality: a systematic review." *ACS Pharmacology & Translational Science* 4, no. 2 (March 11, 2021): 436–51. https://doi .org/10.1021/acsptsci.1c00024.

Zemishlany Z, Aizenberg D, Weizman A. "Subjective effects of MDMA ('Ecstasy') on human sexual function." *European Psychiatry* 16, no. 2 (March 2001): 127–30. https://doi.org/doi: 10.1016/s0924-9338 (01)00550-8.

Zhang J, An S, Hu W, et al. "The neuroprotective properties of *Hericium erinaceus* in glutamate-damaged differentiated PC12 cells and an Alzheimer's disease mouse model." *International Journal of Molecular Sciences* 17, no. 11 (November 1, 2016): 1810. https://doi.org/10.3390/ijms17111810.

Zelfand, Erica, "MDMA Minus the Toxicity: Supplements to Reduce the Risks," Psychedelic Support (February 2023; updated March 2024). https://psychedelic. support/resources/supplements-to-reduce -side-effects-mdma/.

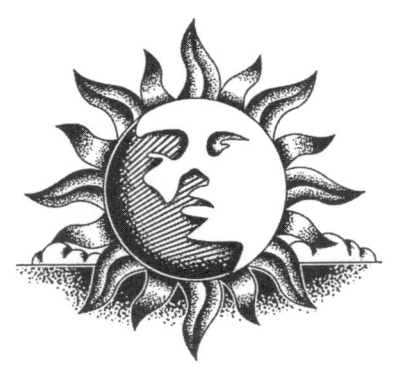

# Index

--------------------

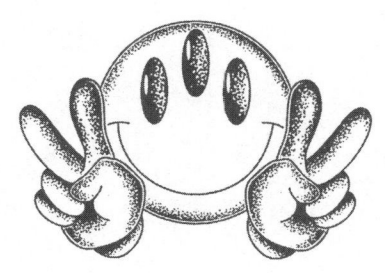